MEDICAL

CW00409223

SCHOOL

A Guide for Teachers

R. H. Trefor Jones, MB, ChB, FRCP(C)

Edward Arnold

A division of Hodder & Stoughton

LONDON BALTIMORE MELBOURNE AUCKLAND

*To my wife Peggy
and our own erstwhile school children
Alyson, Lesley, Valerie, Michael and Trevor.*

Copyright © 1988 R. H. Trefor Jones
First published in Great Britain 1988

British Library Cataloguing in Publication Data

Jones, R. H. Trefor
   Medical conditions in school children: a
   guide for teachers.
   1. Children. Medical aspects—For teaching
   I. Title
   618.92

ISBN 0-7131-7760-8

Typeset by Rowland Phototypesetting Limited,
Bury St Edmunds, Suffolk.
Printed and bound in Great Britain for Edward Arnold, the
educational, academic and medical publishing division of
Hodder and Stoughton Limited, Mill Road, Dunton Green,
Sevenoaks, Kent, by Richard Clay Limited, Bungay, Suffolk.

CONTENTS

INTRODUCTION

This book has been written primarily for teachers in ordinary schools. Its purpose is to outline the more common medical conditions occurring in children which affect their schooling, and to suggest specific guidelines for teachers responsible for the management of such problems in the classroom and the general school environment. I hope it will also be of value to other professionals, such as educational psychologists, social workers, school nurses, health visitors and clinical medical officers who, in their capacity, deal with many children who will have some of the conditions which are referred to, but who may be unaware of the effects certain illnesses have on a child's school work.

It was not my intention to dwell in too great a detail on conditions which one meets in special schools, such as severe physical handicap which require complex educational and other services, but instead to concentrate on those conditions which are encountered in ordinary schools. From the ages of four to sixteen, children spend almost half their waking hours at school. About 10%–15% of these children suffer from illnesses which may affect their academic progress, the relationship they have with their peers and teachers and, in some instances, their physical tolerance. At many stages in their careers teachers will have in their charge a child with such an illness. It is important, therefore, that teachers are familiar with these conditions, how they present, how they are treated, what effect they may have on the child, how the child's education is affected, what steps to take if any problems arise in school and what limitations, if any, are necessary in the child's physical activities.

When dealing with these problems there must be a partnership between teacher, parent and doctor, together with any other agency that may be involved. There should be adequate communication between each individual concerned with the child to ensure that there is a clear understanding of the existing problem and that there is uniformity of approach which can only be beneficial to the child. Without this partnership, and without free communication, each agency acts alone, leading to conflicting advice and misunderstanding which will be to the detriment of children under their care.

In addition to the obvious benefit that cooperation brings to the child, the sharing of responsibility brings parent, teacher and doctor closer together which is an essential partnership in educational medicine so aptly defined in the Court Report *Fit for the Future* as:

> '. . . the study and practice of child health and paediatrics in relation to the process of learning. It requires an understanding of child development, the child's response to schooling, the disorders which interfere with a child's capacity to learn and the specific needs of the handicapped. Its practitioners need to work cooperatively with the teachers, psychologists and others who may be involved with the child and to understand the influence of family and social environment' (HMSO 1978).

Following the 1981 Education Act, based on the recommendations of the Warnock Committee Report, we are witnessing an increasing integration of children with special needs into ordinary schools. This demands a clear understanding on the part of teachers of the disorders and medical problems of school children, and also an even closer partnership between parent, teacher, doctor and other professionals in their management.

GENERAL NOTE FOR TEACHERS

It is important that teachers should be aware of children in their classes who have a known medical condition. Ideally, there should be an opportunity at the beginning of a school year for such conditions to be discussed between the parents and the teachers. Further discussions may be necessary between the teacher and the School Health Service and may involve the child's general practitioner and paediatrician. Close cooperation between the parents, teachers and other professionals involved in the care of the child is essential in order to ensure a clear understanding of the child's illness. This should include details of how the illness may affect the child in school, what academic expectations there may be, what limitations, if any, may be necessary in the child's physical activities, what complications of the condition may occur and how they present, what action should be taken in the event of any complication and how the parents should be contacted. If the child is on any medication, the teacher should be aware of this and be familiar with the possible complications of the treatment which may be noticed in school.

Symptoms of a disorder may arise during the child's schooling and, if this is the case, it is the responsibility of the parents and the School Health Service to inform the teaching staff.

Direct communication between teachers and medical staff may, occasionally, be a problem since any medical information regarding a child can only be relayed with the consent of the parents. Most parents readily agree to this, as it can only be advantageous to the child.

Communication With Parents

Known medical conditions
If a child has a known medical condition (e.g. epilepsy, asthma or diabetes) which may give rise to problems in school, it is essential that teachers know where to contact the child's parents. There should therefore be a record of the parents' home telephone number, or work telephone number if both

parents are working. If this is not possible, the telephone number of a family friend, neighbour, or a relative who can be contacted in an emergency would be valuable.

When speaking to the parents on the telephone, the teacher should remain calm and should stress that the situation is under control. Specific advice which might be helpful in the management of the child should be requested. If a parent is being asked to come to the school, any expression of panic transmitted by the teacher may be upsetting, particularly if a parent intends driving to school, since panic may impair an individual's judgment.

Unexpected emergency

If a child has to be taken from school to hospital for the treatment of an unexpected illness or an injury, it is important to contact the parents as soon as possible. Not only is it important to inform them of the event but, for example, if the child requires surgery the parents' signed consent will be necessary.

It is important to remain calm and reassuring when informing parents of a major incident requiring admission to hospital. If possible the child should be accompanied by a member of staff since this helps to provide comfort and support for the child, and is reassuring to the parents.

Suspected medical conditions

If a teacher suspects that a child has a medical problem it is best to inform the parents in writing. The problem should be outlined, and a suggestion made that the parents seek advice from their general practitioner (taking the teacher's letter with them on their visit). A suspected diagnosis should not be suggested as this could cause unnecessary alarm to the parents.

If no action has been taken as a result of a teacher writing to the parents, the matter should be discussed with the School Health Service. The School Health Service has a responsibility to see and examine the child. They will contact the parents, informing them when the child will be seen and inviting them to be present. Any further arrangements can then be made by the School Health Service doctor.

Suspected problems with treatment

When a child is on treatment for a particular condition, two possible developments may occur. First, the treatment may gradually become less effective and symptoms may start to reappear. Second, the treatment may produce some complications. Parents may not always be aware that the child has any problems since, in some instances, these may only be noticeable in school (e.g. lack of concentration, day-dreaming, sleepiness etc.).

If a teacher notices any change in a child who is known to be on treatment, this should be communicated to the parents by letter, with the suggestion that it should be brought to the attention of their child's doctor. If the teacher is uncertain that the child's problem is related to treatment, this should be discussed with the School Health Service.

It is important that the teacher is aware of the possible complications of some of the commonly used medications, and also what particular features are indicative that the treatment is not as effective as planned.

The Use of Medication in School

Most doctors who treat children are cognisant with the fact that they dislike taking any form of treatment during school hours. The aim of most programmes of preventive treatment is to administer the necessary medication at home. In some conditions this is not possible. With epilepsy, for example, in order to maintain an adequate blood level of some anti-epileptic drugs, it is necessary for the child to take a tablet or medicine at midday. Since it is not always possible for the child to go home at lunch time, the medication will have to be given at school. Although most children, particularly in secondary schools, are capable of taking their own treatment, some schools prefer that this is supervised by a teacher. This will vary depending on the child, the treatment, and the regulations pertaining in some Local Education Authorities.

If any problems exist in a particular school with respect to the administration of medication, it is advisable for this to be discussed by the headteacher, parents and the doctor supervising the child's treatment so that a satisfactory compromise can be worked out.

Ideally, most schools, particularly the larger secondary schools, should have a school nurse as a permanent member of staff, who is able to supervise such treatment and who would also be involved with health education, talks on drug and alcohol abuse, parenthood classes and, in addition, would provide a first aid service for the school. However, although such posts were recommended in the Court Report, few appointments have been made.

School Day Trips

Day trips from school have become a regular feature of school life and are educational and enjoyable. It is unnecessary to exclude a child who has medical problems from these events but, in some instances, certain precautions will have to be taken. (See under separate headings: epilepsy, diabetes, asthma.)

School Outings Abroad

Schools are increasingly taking groups of children abroad for periods of educational and sporting activities. There can be no blanket rule concerning the participation of children with medical problems on such tours. Each child will have to be considered individually with respect to the particular condition and its severity, the likelihood of any problems arising, the attitude of the child and the parents, the experience of the teacher supervising the group and the ease of availability of emergency treatment should it become necessary.

When a child with a known medical condition goes abroad with a school group, the supervising teacher should be familiar with the child's condition. This should include an awareness of any likely complications, appropriate treatment, medication to be taken, how to contact the parents, where help can be obtained in the region being visited and how the child's doctor can be reached.

Most children who have conditions which are likely to present problems carry an identification disc in the form of a necklace or a bracelet. Each disc will be inscribed with the child's particular registration number and the telephone number of the hospital or doctor which the child normally attends. It is rarely necessary to preclude a child's involvement in a school visit abroad. Diabetic children, for example, are extremely self-reliant and are often more familiar with their treatment and diet than their parents. Likewise, children with asthma are frequently better in the dry, fresh air of a skiing resort than they are at home.

Moving Schools

When a child moves from a junior to a senior school or moves to a school in another locality, it is important that information regarding the child's medical condition is relayed to the new school. The School Health Service maintains records on every school child which contain details of diagnosis and treatment. When a child transfers from one school to another such information is available through them to the teaching staff.

When a child moves away from the area, the school health records are transferred to the District Community Physician in the new location. Similar transfers of medical records occur from the family doctor to the new family doctor. Unfortunately, such transfers may take a few weeks and it is therefore important that the parents are advised to inform the child's new school of any problems the child has. It is also advisable for them to register immediately with a family doctor of their choice in their new locality.

ABDOMINAL PAIN

Prevalence

Abdominal pain occurring in a child at school is probably one of the most frequent and one of the most difficult problems encountered by teachers. Even after a medical examination, the exact nature of abdominal pain is, in many children, not easily ascertained. In general, there are two presentations of abdominal pain: one occurring suddenly in a child who has had no previous episode, and one occurring in a child who has pain periodically.

ACUTE PAIN

Any child who presents to the teacher with acute abdominal pain, and who has not previously complained, should be treated seriously. Arrangements should be made with the parents for the child to be collected from school and taken to the family doctor. In a residential school, the child should be admitted to the sick room and kept in bed until the arrival of the school doctor. Nothing should be given orally to the child before the doctor arrives.

The primary diagnosis to be considered is one of acute appendicitis. In the early stages, examination may not reveal the diagnosis and the child may have to be seen again an hour or two later, to be re-examined.

An infection of the intestines (enteritis) may also present in a similar way with acute abdominal pain or colic. This is usually accompanied by diarrhoea and also, occasionally, by vomiting. The child should be sent home or, if in a residential school, isolated.

RECURRENT, NON-ORGANIC PAIN

Many children complain of recurrent abdominal pain without there being any obvious underlying cause. This often occurs in children during the first year or two of schooling. It is usually short in duration and frequently disappears if the child's attention is diverted. Recurrent, non-organic abdominal pain seems to become more frequent as the child becomes older and reaches a peak at about the age of nine. Girls are more commonly affected than boys.

This type of pain is often associated with pallor and occasionally, nausea and vomiting. Its close relation to migraine gives rise to the term, used by some, 'abdominal migraine'. The child tends to be rather quiet, often withdrawn, conscientious and of average or above average intelligence. There is sometimes a tendency to strive to achieve a higher educational standard than the child is intellectually capable of. It is therefore assumed that stress plays an important part in the cause of the child's symptoms. Although the underlying cause may, in part, be psychological, the pain itself is real and can be compared to headaches adults suffer from after a stressful day.

It is difficult to generalise regarding the advice to be given in this situation, since any action will vary depending on the individual child, the child's response to pain and the frequency of attacks and their severity. Many children who suffer this type of pain are able to continue their normal activities, but others will report to the teacher every time they experience pain. Some will have pain only prior to a particular stressful situation (e.g. examinations). In a small number of children, abdominal pain will commence before they leave the house for school. This may cause them to be kept at home, although, the pain itself will often go in a short while.

In the first instance, the teacher should attempt to reassure the child, particularly if in previous experience the duration of the pain has been short. Helping the child to relax and talk through anxieties and stress associated with school work also alleviates the situation. Occasionally, despite every effort by the teacher, the child may have to be taken home.

See also   Cystitis, Diarrhoea and Vomiting, Dysmenorrhoea, Hepatitis, School Refusal

AIDS (ACQUIRED IMMUNODEFICIENCY SYNDROME)

AIDS is rarely seen in children, and occurs due to an abnormal response of the body to infection by the human immunodeficiency virus (HIV). The condition is characterised by a higher than normal incidence of infections, loss of weight and certain skin cancers.

AIDS is confined mainly to two groups of children. The first group is newborn babies who have acquired HIV infection by transmission from an infected mother during pregnancy and in whom the disease is rapidly fatal. The second group is boys who have haemophilia and who have become accidentally infected by HIV contaminated blood products given during treatment. (*See* Haemophilia.)

In view of the possible risk of social isolation that may occur if a child is known to be infected with HIV, it is important that the number of people, including teachers, who are aware of this should be confined only to those who need to know in order that they may ensure the proper care of the child. Because a child with AIDS has a reduced resistance to even the more common childhood infections, he/she may require longer periods of absence from school to recover.

Risk Situations

Some situations may arise in school where there is a risk of transmission of the virus and it is therefore important to observe certain precautions. The more likely risk situations are:

1 *External bleeding*

– Follow normal first-aid procedures and, if possible, wear rubber gloves.
– A wound should be washed with soap and water and covered with a large waterproof dressing.

- A nose bleed should be controlled by cold compress pressure.
- Seek medical advice as soon as possible.
- Contaminated towels, dressings or gloves should be 'double bagged' in yellow bags and arrangements for incineration made with the local authority.
- Contaminated clothing should be washed in a machine at 95°C for ten minutes before washing normally.

2 Contamination of another person

If there is any contamination of any other person or a child with blood from a known HIV-positive child, it should be dealt with as follows:

- The skin should be washed copiously with soap and water.
- The eyes should be irrigated copiously with water.
- Any laceration in a person who is likely to deal with an HIV positive child should be covered by a waterproof dressing.

3 Personal hygiene and practices

- Toothbrushes and razors should not be shared.
- Ear piercing should be carried out only at recognised establishments using disposable or sterilised equipment.
- Tattooing of school children by each other should be actively discouraged. (It is an offence to tattoo a child under the age of sixteen years.)
- The making of 'blood brothers' by the mingling of blood, following cutting or pricking the skin, should be actively discouraged.

No Risk

To date, there is no evidence that there is any risk of transmission of HIV infection from:

1 Droplet infection – such as sneezing, coughing or spitting.
2 Normal social contact.
3 Sharing eating or drinking utensils.
4 Sharing washing and showering facilities.
5 Sharing musical instruments.
6 Using normal swimming pools (i.e. chlorinated pools).

School Activities

A child who is HIV positive should be allowed to participate in any school activity which his/her medical condition allows. The normal safety precautions that pertain to such events as woodwork, metal work and craft should be observed.

Further detailed publications on AIDS are available from the Department of Education and Science, Welsh Office Information Division and the Health Education Council – the addresses of which appear at the back of the book.

ALCOHOL

The apparent earlier physical maturity of today's adolescents, coupled with the irregular enforcement of drinking laws and the easy availability of alcoholic beverages in supermarkets has resulted in an increase in heavy drinking among young children. The ready acceptance of alcohol in society and in the home enhances this further.

In general, the younger children are when they start regular social drinking, the more problems they encounter in their relationship with society. Regular bouts of drinking in a school child produce deterioration of school work and frequent absences from school for alleged illnesses. There is often depression or remorse after drinking bouts and behavioural changes.

By identifying and confirming the existence of alcoholism in an adolescent, the teacher is obliged, at an early age, to involve the parents. It is hoped that the parents will share the teacher's concern. Unfortunately, children who have drinking problems frequently have parents who themselves are alcoholics. The young alcoholics and heavy drinkers also tend to have a very poor relationship with their parents.

In view of the frequently-present personality disorders resulting from a mixture of genetics and environment, the results of counselling and treatment are, unfortunately, disappointing. Much of the treatment should be directed towards containment of the problem until the adolescent eventually matures. Occasionally, group therapy and individual psychotherapy may be necessary, hence referral to the School Psychological Service and Child Guidance Clinic would be advisable.

ALLERGY

Allergy is probably the most common of all childhood conditions and produces a variety of different symptoms and illnesses.

An allergic reaction is an abnormal response by the body to a substance (an allergen) that an individual is sensitive to. The reaction only occurs in certain susceptible individuals and the reason for this, and the actual mechanism involved, is not clearly understood. Many factors are responsible and the allergens can be either inhaled or ingested, producing different reactions from one child to another. Examples of inhaled allergens are pollen, animal dander and fur, house dust, house dust mite, feathers and moulds. Examples of ingested allergens are eggs, milk, citrus fruit, fish and nuts.

An allergic reaction may manifest itself in different ways, either by a rash (urticaria or eczema), a runny nose, runny red eyes (hay fever – allergic rhinitis or allergic conjunctivitis), a more severe reaction with swelling of the eyes and lips (angioneurotic oedema) or wheezing (asthma). (*See also* Eczema and Asthma.)

URTICARIA

Presentation

Urticaria (or hives) is recognised by the presence of an intermittent, raised, red blotchy rash with a pale centre which is intensely itchy. The lesions vary in size and can be from ½ in to 1 in in diameter. They are similar in appearance to a nettle sting.

Cause

The exact allergen which causes urticaria in childhood is frequently not established. Most are thought to be due to an ingested allergen and occasionally, there may be a clear history of urticaria occurring within a few hours of a certain food having been eaten, which makes the diagnosis easier. In the majority of children, further tests are necessary in order to attempt to establish the causative agent.

In some children, an urticarial rash occurs when they are exposed to cold conditions (e.g. after coming out of the swimming pool). In this instance, the rash disappears after a warm shower.

Treatment

The treatment is directed, if possible, at avoiding the known allergens. Failing this, the rash responds to treatment with oral antihistamines such as Piriton, Phenergan or Vallergan, which have usually been prescribed by the child's medical practitioner.

If a child is subject to frequent attacks of urticaria, the availability of such antihistamines for an individual child in school would be an advantage since early treatment is helpful. A child whose urticaria is more troublesome may require treatment on a daily basis. Since one of the side effects of antihistamines is drowsiness, a preparation such as Triludan, which produces less drowsiness, may be used.

SEVERE ALLERGY (ANGIO-NEUROTIC OEDEMA)

Presentation

In this condition, there is a sudden onset of swelling of the tissues surrounding the eyes and of the lips with or without urticaria. This may occur in any child without there being a previous history of allergy. It is a potentially dangerous situation since the swelling may involve the tongue and the tissues of the pharynx which may impede the child's breathing.

Treatment

Urgent treatment is necessary and the child should be taken immediately to the nearest hospital emergency department.

HAY FEVER

Presentation

Hay fever is characterised by frequent sneezing, an itchy and runny nose and red, itchy eyes. It occurs more commonly during the early summer when the pollen count is highest.

The symptoms of hay fever are often quite severe and may be associated with generalised lassitude. Since these symptoms occur at a time of year when most of the important examinations take place, children who suffer from hay fever are frequently at a disadvantage.

Cause

The most common cause is an allergy to grass pollen but any of the common pollens may be factors. The symptoms may be aggravated by other allergens or irritants such as house dust, chalk dust or animal fur.

Treatment

Avoidance of pollen is impossible and the only measures that can be taken are:

1 Not to play in fields that have been recently mowed.
2 Not to handle furry animals in the classroom.
3 To keep out of dusty areas such as classrooms that are being cleaned.
4 To use damp dusting of blackboards.

Specific treatment necessitates the use of antihistamines such as Piriton, Phenergan or Vallergan. If they need to be given on a daily basis, and particularly if they cause drowsiness, a preparation such as Triludan may be used. Other preparations which are used for the treatment of hay fever are nasal drops or sprays containing disodium cromoglycate (trade name, Rynacrom) which blocks the allergic response and hence reduces the nasal obstruction and watery discharge. More severe cases may require the use of cortisone preparations such as a

Beconase spray. In children who have accompanying red and irritable eyes (allergic conjuctivitis), similar preparations may be necessary as eye drops.

Courses of desensitisation injections of graduated concentrations of pollen have been used in the past but, in view of their potential dangers, these are now rarely prescribed.

See also   Asthma, Eczema, Migraine

ANAEMIA

Anaemia is the most common blood disorder seen in children. It is characterised by pallor and tiredness. There are numerous causes of anaemia which may result from either imperfect red blood cells or an inadequate number being formed.

IRON DEFICIENCY ANAEMIA

In order to function effectively, each red cell requires an adequate level of the chemical haemoglobin. Haemoglobin is responsible for the transportation of oxygen from the lungs to the tissues, and carbon dioxide from the tissues to the lungs. One of the most important elements necessary for the formation of haemoglobin is iron.

The dietary intake of iron may be deficient as a result of a poor appetite or a diet low in iron, such as in a strict vegetarian or vegan diet. Some children develop a habit of eating only a high carbohydrate diet consisting mainly of milk, bread, cereals and biscuits, all of which are low in iron.

In addition to pallor and tiredness, common to other causes of anaemia, children with iron deficiency are irritable and have a very poor appetite. The latter may add further to an already low intake of iron.

In rare instances, iron deficiency anaemia can occur as a result of blood loss or in certain parasitic infections such as hookworm.

Treatment

Before treatment begins any other possible causative factor must be ruled out.

One of the most important aspects of treatment is directed at maintaining a balanced diet and hence, dietary education in school plays a vital role. Children with food fads and poor dietary habits occasionally require admission to hospital for observation and advice before they revert to eating a normal diet.

There are many iron preparations which are used for replacement treatment and because only a small amount of iron in any preparation is absorbed, they have to be given at least two or three times daily. This means that they may occasionally have to be administered in school. Because certain foods, particularly milk and cereal, interfere with the absorption of iron, medication has to be given between meals. Since liquid preparations can stain the teeth of a child, administration should be followed by vigorousy brushing the teeth.

HAEMOLYTIC ANAEMIAS

These anaemias are caused by excessive damage of the red blood cells, either due to an abnormality of the wall of the cells or because of defective formation and instability of the chemical haemoglobin inside the cells. (*See* Sickle Cell Disease and Thalassaemia.)

DEFECTIVE PRODUCTION OF RED CELLS

In some extremely rare congenital conditions, the bone marrow is only able to produce a low level of red blood cells. A similar result may occur because of certain chemical damage to the bone marrow or because of the infiltration of bone marrow with abnormal tissue. (*See* Leukaemia.)

See also   Sickle Cell Disease, Thalassaemia, Leukaemia (Acute)

ANOREXIA NERVOSA

This is an exceedingly rare condition in childhood. When it does occur, it is usually during the adolescent period and is almost entirely confined to girls.

The development of anorexia nervosa usually follows a similar pattern. The child is generally a pubertal or post-pubertal girl who started off by being overweight, or who thought of herself as being overweight, and consequently started dieting. Weight loss is usually achieved by following diets seen in teenage magazines or simply by limiting almost all food intake. Such a child may have a mother who is over-weight and consequently diets as a precaution in case she too follows a similar trend.

Although some girls with this condition are honest regarding their reduced food intake, most conceal this fact and exaggerate or lie about the amount they are eating. Despite their weight loss and their poor diet most children who have anorexia nervosa are physically active, healthy and intelligent and make good progress at school. As the condition progresses there may well be damage to the child's health and death from starvation or a severe coincidental infection can occur.

Emotional disturbances in children with anorexia nervosa are common and, therefore, the condition is best handled by a psychiatrist. Regular counselling will be necessary with the child and family, and occasionally it may be necessary for the child to be admitted into hospital for closer supervision and treatment.

ASTHMA

Prevalence

It is estimated that asthma occurs in about 5% of all school children. As a single chronic condition, it causes a higher percentage of days lost from school than any other disease.

Presentation

Asthma is characertised by recurrent attacks of coughing, breathlessness and wheezing. The symptoms arise at varying intervals and are of differing degrees of severity and may be brought about by any of the following:

– respiratory infection;
– allergy;
– emotional stress;
– a combination of any or all of the first three factors.

In addition, milder episodes of wheezing may be precipitated by exercise or exposure to cold and windy conditions in some children.

Many of the attacks from which a child suffers in school are mild; others require rest for a short period of time, perhaps after taking appropriate medication. Occasionally, the child may have a paroxysm of uncontrollable coughing. If this does not pass in a short while, the use of the same medication may alleviate the spasm. The child should not be sent out for a glass of water as in some instances this may aggravate the cough. Certain classroom activities can produce sufficient respiratory irritation to precipitate coughing and wheezing. Examples are: dry dusting of the blackboard, dry sweeping of floors, stuffy and poorly ventilated rooms and animals kept in the classroom.

Much has been written in the past concerning the personality traits of children with asthma but, in a condition with such a varying degree of severity, there will be an equal variety of personality differences. Asthmatic children are often said to be anxious, dependent and immature. The anxiety is understandable but, like many features, seems to be present only in a child with severe symptoms. Dependency will be present if there is excessive and needless over-protection by the parents – again, more likely a feature of severe asthma. Immaturity may arise as a result of over-protection. However, the majority of children with asthma have normal behaviour and personality.

Additional features are said to be lack of self-confidence, latent aggression, depression and egocentricity. However, observers are more likely to recall children with abnormal traits than they are those with normal behaviour. Prospective studies have been carried out on asthmatic children with specific regard to personality, school achievement and IQ. These studies have demonstrated that personality abnormalities are rare and occur only in those with severe symptoms. The average IQ is slightly highter than in the general child population.

ACUTE ASTHMA ATTACK

Severe attacks of asthma are heralded by increasing breathlessness, wheezing and marked difficulty in exhaling. The child becomes distressed and anxious and there is an accompanying increase in the respiratory and pulse rate. If the attack is very severe, the child's lips and finger nails may become blue.

Calmness and constant reassurance is essential when dealing with such a situation since any anxiety displayed by the teacher is easily transmitted to the child. The usual medication that the child needs for such an attack should always be available and should be used in an attempt to relieve the symptoms. It is important that the recommended dosages are not exceeded.

In the event of a severe attack, the parents, general practitioner, or school doctor should be contacted immediately so that arrangements regarding further treatment can be made.

Treatment

The severity of the child's asthma will dictate the medication used, the mode of administration and the frequency with which it is given. Treatment will be considered under three headings: avoidance, prevention and specific drugs.

Avoidance

Most children with asthma will have had specific tests carried out to determine what, if anything, they are allergic to. These tests take the form of either skin tests, using specific extracts of the more common allergens, or blood tests where the levels of certain antibodies are measured. Often the association between asthma and an allergen is already known to the child because of previous experience.

The child will therefore have to avoid all the factors to which he/she is allergic. The commonest are: house dust, house dust mite, animal fur or dander, feathers, pollen, grass, and certain foods. In the classroom, the child should not be seated too near the blackboard because of dust, or too near any animals that may be present.

Prevention

Certain preventive medications are taken on a regular basis to prevent attacks from occurring. These are:

1 *Intal (disodium cromoglycate)*

This is administered either by means of a spinhaler (a device for delivering the contents of a capsule containing Intal into the lungs by forced inhalations) or by means of an atomised spray. This may need to be given at school as it should be used three or four times daily.

2 *Slophylline*
   Uniphylline

These are oral preparations in which the effective component is slowly released into the blood stream. They are usually only given once or twice daily and will rarely need to be given at school.

3 *Becotide*
   Pulmicort

These are both cortisone derivatives and are used in children with moderate to severe asthma. They are administered by means of an atomiser.

4   *Prednisone*
     Prednisolone

These are oral cortisone preparations which are used occasionally in children with severe asthma.

Specific drugs

Despite much improvement in preventive treatment, attacks of asthma will still occur and treatment of these may be needed in school. The agents more commonly used are:

Ventolin (Salbutamol)
Briconyl (Terbutaline)
Bronchodil (Reproterol)

In order to obtain immediate results, the agents are usually administered by means of an atomiser. The dosage to be given, and the frequency, should be ascertained from the parents since it is dangerous to exceed the recommended dosage. On rare occasions a child may become almost addicted to the use of an atomised spray which is reflected by an increase in self-administration. If this is suspected the matter should be reported to the child's parents.

As will be mentioned later, in order not to wheeze, some children require the use of these agents before they undertake any physical activity. This group of drugs, known as bronchodilators, can also be given by syrup or tablet form, if the effect needs to be more prolonged.

Physical Activity

Children who have asthma should not be excluded from any sport or physical activity for which they have the necessary training and skill. Asthmatic children should, in fact, be actively encouraged to participate as exercise is beneficial rather than detrimental to their health. The form of activity will depend in great part on their interest and ability, although it should be recognised that intermittent exercise is less provocative than a continuous one. Patterns of running, which are part of most ball games, are well tolerated. At the same time, the selection of a child for a team, on merit, will be a major achievement for both the child and the family.

In a child with moderate to severe asthma, there may occasionally be some residual chest deformity and, associated with this, poor thoracic muscle development. If this is the case, then the following activities should be encouraged: weight lifting, canoeing, rowing, karate, judo, wrestling, and swimming.

A warm up period immediately prior to participation in sport is very important for a child with asthma. It should take the form of a moderate exercise programme lasting at least five minutes. This may well reduce the possibility of exercise-induced wheezing because of the gradual release of chemical mediators by the body. It also serves a useful purpose (as it does in any child) since:

- it reduces the risk of injury;
- it assists limb and joint flexibility; and
- it enhances skill and performance.

In practice, this period will often alleviate mild wheezing or tightness of the chest.

Swimming is probably one of the best forms of exercise and sport for asthmatic children to participate in. They should also be encouraged to pursue this after school hours. Swimming is less likely to provoke exercise-induced asthma than any other activity. Occasionally, the high chlorine content of some swimming pools produces wheezing in a small number of children. This may be overcome by the use of preventive treatment.

Track and field events can be encouraged, with the possible exception of long distance running, particularly in cold weather.

Pre-exercise Treatment

Because exercise may produce wheezing in some children, it is perfectly reasonable to use an agent that will reduce or prevent this symptom from occurring. This has now become more generally recognised and many well-known athletes and sportsmen and women use such agents prior to participating in an event. For example, in the 1980 Olympics, each of the three

25

Australian asthmatics who won medals (two gold in swimming and one silver in track athletics) required medication before their events.

The medication to be used should be delivered by means of an atomiser immediately before the activity occurs. All treatment takes about 45 minutes to work effectively. In the case of international competitions which are subject to doping controls, the medication used must be on the approved list of the Medical Commission of the International Olympic Committee.

Other Activities

An asthmatic child may play any wind instrument. This has never been found to be harmful and may encourage breath control. Active encouragement should therefore be given to asthmatic children to participate in almost any physical activity in school. There is almost no sport that they cannot take part in, and their involvement not only helps to improve their condition physically but also gives them the emotional satisfaction of leading a normal school life.

See also   Allergy

ATAXIA – *see* Cerebral Palsy

ATHETOSIS – *see* Cerebral Palsy

ATHLETE'S FOOT

The infection which causes athletes foot is due to a fungus, usually an epidermophyton or trichophyton fungus. Transmission of the fungus is through water contact in showers and swimming pools, or through infected shoes or socks.

Presentation

There is intense itching on the soles of the feet and on the skin between the toes. The skin becomes red, scaly and breaks down.

Prevention

1 Disinfected foot baths should be strictly used before and after children use the swimming pool.
2 There should be adequate showering facilities after games and swimming, and disinfectant treatment of floors in the shower room and cubicles.
3 Early detection of the problem with early referral for treatment will reduce the risk of any infection spreading.

Treatment

The agent used is Clotrimazole which is available as a solution, cream, spray, or powder. It is best to use a solution or spray for direct application, but the powder should be used only for the treatment of shoes and socks.

ATTENTION DEFICIT DISORDER

This was, at one time, referred to as minimal brain damage, but because of the implications of the words 'brain damage' a much more satisfactory name is attention deficit disorder with or without hyperactivity. The child with an attention deficit disorder is of normal intelligence, but has behavioural or learning problems. These manifest themselves as a short attention span, impaired memory, poor language comprehension and poor verbal self-expression. The child will therefore exhibit difficulty in understanding instructions, organising his/her work and completing assigned tasks. Because of the defects in abstract thinking, memory and communication, the child is often thought to be lazy and inattentive. Restlessness may be present if the child is also hyperactive.

Children with this disorder require teaching in a small group with almost individual instruction. They require firm and consistent handling and avoidance of abstract teaching. Early advice and assessment by an educational psychologist with a view to appropriate placement will be necessary.

BLINDNESS – *see* Visual Handicap

CEREBRAL PALSY

The term 'cerebral palsy' is a wide one and encompasses all the conditions where there is a disordered movement of the body or limbs due to underlying disease or damage of part of the brain. The type of movement disorder will depend on the part of the brain affected, and the severity will depend on the amount of damage or disease present.

Presentation

A child with cerebral palsy may have very loose or floppy muscles (hypotonia), a finding which is common in very young children. On the other hand, the muscles may be very stiff or tight (hypertonia). The term spastic refers also to the tightness of the muscles. Usually a child with cerebral palsy has associated handicaps, such as hearing and visual defects, perceptual problems and also learning difficulties of differing degrees. The incidence of cerebral palsy is 2.5 per 1000 population.

HEMIPLEGIA

This type of cerebral palsy results in a paralysis or weakness of the arm and leg on one side of the body. It is responsible for 30% of the total cases of cerebral palsy. A right hemiplegia occurs in 70% of the children affected. In 60% of all cases, the intelligence is normal or near normal.

The arm of a child with hemiplegia is held in a characteristic position. The hand is kept closed forming a fist and both elbow and wrist are bent or flexed. Often there is also a tendency for the shoulder to turn inwards. The grasp of the hand is weak and there is an inability to perform intricate movements of the fingers. There is difficulty in recognising shapes and texture by touch. The leg is flexed at the hip and knee and turned slightly inwards. The child walks on the toes with the foot extended at the ankle. The affected leg and arm have poorer circulation than the normal limbs and hence, feel colder to the touch, and there is an overall reduction in size of the affected side.

Despite having normal intelligence, these children have considerable educational problems due mainly to specific learning disorders. Reading delay and number difficulties occur in 60% of hemiplegic children with normal intelligence.

DIPLEGIA

This type of cerebral palsy is present when the muscle weakness and tightness or spasticity is greater in both legs than in the arms. The resulting muscle tightness causes difficulty in walking, which is executed by a waddling, stiff gait. The tightness also causes the legs to become crossed or scissored.

If the legs are predominantly involved, the child's intelligence is much nearer normal, but there may still be associated severe learning problems. Even in the absence of any grossly obvious changes in the arms, there may be difficulty learning skilled manipulation.

QUADREPLEGIA

In this condition there is muscle weakness and tightness involving all four limbs.

ATAXIA

Ataxia occurs because of disease or damage to the part of the brain (the cerebellum) which coordinates information concerning muscle movement. As a consequence, the child is unable to control the speed, strength, or direction of a simple movement. This results in an unsteady drunken gait with the feet held widely apart for balance. Incoordinate movement of the hand causes difficulty in writing and in performing intricate tasks.

DISORDERED MOVEMENT (DYSKINESIA)

One group of children with cerebral palsy have a disorder of movement. This results in involuntary movements of the face, limbs, or body, with associated abnormality of muscle tone. It occurs because of a disorder or disease in part of the cerebrum which receives information from all the other parts of the brain concerning execution or plan of movement (i.e. the force, the direction and the position of parts of the body or the body itself in space) in relation to vision and balance.

The two main types of disordered movement are chorea and athetosis. The distinction between them is a fine one and they may co-exist, hence they are often considered together as choreo-athetosis.

CHOREA

The involuntary movements in chorea result in unpredictable and sudden jerking of the arms and head. The child is often restless and fidgety and choreoform movements of the face cause constant grimacing. The movements are exaggerated when the child becomes excited. The lips, tongue and palate are involved so that feeding and speech may be difficult. The jerking movements of the head and arms are much more exaggerated than those in the trunk and legs. During sleep or periods of relaxation, the movements may disappear.

ATHETOSIS

The movements in athetosis are slower and result in a more gradual change of posture. The upper limbs are constantly moving and there is also grimacing and movement of the face and tongue and, as in chorea, there is difficulty with feeding and with speech.

Associated Problems of Cerebral Palsy

The relatively small number of children with cerebral palsy educated at ordinary schools are the groups with hemiplegia and diplegia, where there is fairly normal intelligence, some learning problems and reasonable mobility. Many children, therefore, require placement at special schools, mainly because of the associated problems that co-exist with cerebral palsy and a consequent need for therapy and for alternative methods of education. Associated problems which occur are:

Speech defects
Speech problems are particularly common in children with

choreo-athetosis and early help with speech therapy is essential. The speech may continue to remain so indistinct that the child requires other means of communication. This may be sign language (Paget Gorman), special symbols (Bliss Symbolics) that can be indicated to by eye, head or hand movement, or by specially adapted, illuminated letter and number screens attached to typewriters which the child can operate by means of a trigger which can be modified to suit each individual (Possum). Finally, more sophisticated methods of communication are now available using computers with a printout facility.

Special educational problems

Because of the difficulties with concepts of space, shape and direction in most children with cerebral palsy, there is a major perceptual problem. This causes reading, writing and numeracy difficulties and, when present in a child who has concomitantly a short attention span, they raise considerable educational problems. These problems may be present despite the fact that the child has fairly normal intelligence.

Mobility

Apart from the group with hemiplegia and some who have diplegia, mobility is a problem for the majority of the other affected children. Almost all will require frequent physiotherapy to prevent muscle contracture and to encourage movement and weight-bearing. Weight-bearing is important even in a child who spends all day in a wheelchair, since it is necessary for transferring them from chair to bed, or chair to toilet. In addition, a certain amount of daily weight-bearing reduces the risk of loss of bone calcium.

Special chairs require space for operation, ramps, wider doorways and facilities for battery charging. Instructions for the use of wheelchairs and maintenance of proficiency is also essential. Most schools dealing specifically with cerebral palsy have heated hydrotherapy pools which are used for both limb exercise and enjoyment.

Social problems

Children with choreo-athetosis and some with severe spasticity will require help with feeding and many will also require help with toileting.

Epilepsy

This occurs in between 25%–50% of children affected by cerebral palsy and therapy may have to be administered in school on a regular basis. (*See* Epilepsy)

CHICKEN POX

A child with chicken pox may have very little in the way of constitutional symptoms. The characteristic rash appears in crops over a period of 2 to 7 days. Initially, the lesions are discrete, itchy red spots of about 2 mm in diameter, which appear predominantly on the trunk. Within the first 24 hours, small yellowish-white blisters form on the lesions. Eventually, the blisters rupture and form a crust.

Transmission

Chicken pox is highly infectious and is transmitted by direct contact with an ill child by droplet infection (e.g. from coughing) or less frequently, by airborne transmission.

Incubation Period

The incubation period (from contact to appearance of the illness) is normally from 14 to 16 days but this can vary from 10 to 21 days.

Infectious Period

Chicken pox is infectious and the illness can be transmitted from the day before the rash appears to 5 to 6 days after the blisters have crusted.

CHILD ABUSE

The terms 'child abuse', 'non-accidental injury' or the 'battered child syndrome' are synonymous, and refer to the deliberate injury to a child by a parent or other person in the same household. The battered child syndrome was originally described in 1868 by Ambroise Tardieu, who was a professor of legal medicine in Paris. He described 32 children who had been burnt or battered to death. In 1946, a radiologist from the United States, Dr John Caffey, described bone changes found in children who also had evidence of chronic haemorrhage into the skull. The significance of this as being evidence of repeated trauma was subsequently recognised.

Child abuse does not only relate to physical violence to a child, but also covers physical or emotional neglect and emotional or sexual abuse. Although it is recognised that child abuse occurs more commonly in pre-school children, there is little doubt that many cases occur in older children and may well be noted by an alert teacher.

Prevalence

It is estimated that the NSPCC alone deals with between 25,000 and 30,000 cases annually, involving a total of about 90,000 children. The incidence of actual physical violence is about 4500 cases per year. Of this number, 10%–17% of children will die from their injuries, and 30% will develop physical and/or mental handicap because of brain damage. There are doubtless numerous other cases that are not obvious, in particular those involving emotional abuse and sexual exploitation.

Presentation

The teacher has an important role in the recognition of some of the signs evident in child abuse and, in a proven case, should be involved with planning the child's rehabilitation and supervision. Although many of the features are similar at differing ages, it is convenient to consider the children in two groups: those of nursery or pre-school age and those who are older.

NURSERY AGE CHILDREN

Physical evidence

- Repeated, unexplained injury.
- Scattered bruising found in unusual places.
- Bruising of ear lobes.
- Bruising involving both eyes.
- Suspiciously-shaped bruising (e.g. belt, hand or other instrument).
- Cuts behind ear lobes or inside lips.
- Associated poor nutritional state.

Emotional state

- Withdrawn and quiet child.
- Worried, open eyed expression.
- Often shows little or no emotion.
- Delayed intellectual development.
- Occasionally hyperactive, negative and aggressive.

The last state listed above may be used by parents as an excuse for smacking as the child, in their opinion, cannot be controlled in any other way. This type of behaviour, however, may be the result of physical abuse rather than the cause of it.

OLDER CHILDREN

Physical evidence

There is less opportunity for the teacher to observe evidence of physical abuse in an older child than in a very young one. The features, when present, are the same – however, the older child often attempts to hide any bruising, either by wearing inappropriate clothing, or by avoiding activities such as sport or swimming which necessitate the change of clothing in the presence of other pupils or staff members. Older children may also fabricate stories to explain their injuries, either to protect their parents, or because of threats of further battering should they reveal that their parents were responsible.

Emotional state

- Lonely and friendless.
- Often withdrawn and sullen.
- Occasionally aggressive and hyperactive.
- Poor school performance, particularly in reading and writing.

Often such children, when asked to carry out a specific task, will exhibit such a degree of anxiety as to disorganise their attempt completely. When asked specific questions, the child might feign ignorance rather than risk disapproval of an incorrect answer. The child is often so concerned with the questioner's possible intention that concentration on the question itself is not possible.

ADOLESCENT

The features found in the older child are also found in the adolescent, but this group is more likely to exhibit other abnormal behavioural responses. Adolescents who are subjected to physical abuse at home may run away, yet may not seek help from any other agency and will rarely mention the reason for their wanting to leave home. Occasionally, they find a need to express their anger outside the home and this results in involvement with vandalism and delinquency. Group activities, such as gangs, satisfy the needs of an adolescent who is emotionally deprived by giving him/her a sense of belonging and security. This secure environment further enables them to discharge their aggression.

Action by Teacher

It is well to remember that not every child with multiple bruising has been physically abused and that there are medical reasons why some children bruise easily. In view of this, the initial action taken by the teacher will depend on the degree of suspicion and the presence, or otherwise, of additional factors.

If a child presents with unexplained bruising, the first step would be to discuss the matter with the headteacher and the school nurse or doctor. If, upon examination, the appearance is not suspicious, the school health service should contact the child's parents and arrange for appropriate investigations to be carried out through the family doctor or hospital children's department. If the examination findings of the school doctor or nurse are highly suspicious, contact should be established with the family doctor, or directly with the hospital children's department, to arrange the child's admission for investigation. Simultaneously, there should be direct communication between the headteacher and the local Director of Social Services who has the responsibility of coordinating the other agencies involved and for arranging a case conference.

If a child who has multiple bruising or other evidence of physical abuse admits to a teacher that these are the results of injury inflicted by a parent or other person in the child's household, the matter should be immediately reported to the headteacher. On receiving such information, the headteacher should contact the Director of Social Services and the Community Physician to arrange subsequent action.

Non-accidental Injury Procedure

As a result of problems which have arisen in the past, due to poor communication between the many agencies that may be involved with child abuse, each District Social Services Department has established a recommended procedure to be followed in each case. Although there are slight differences in procedure in some areas, the fundamental principles are the same.

Upon receiving information that a child has been subjected to physical abuse, or that there is evidence giving rise to a high degree of suspicion, the Director of Social Services, through his/her officers, will arrange a case conference. Case conferences are usually arranged within three days of this information being received. Representatives of the agencies that have been, or may be, involved with the child and family, are invited to attend. These may include the general practitioner, health visitor, paediatrician, children's ward sister, social worker, teacher, educational welfare officer, police liaison officer, NSPCC officer and occasionally, a probation officer and local housing officer. The initial purpose of the case conference is to establish the facts concerning the child and family, as known to each agency. Following the sharing of this information, a decision has to be reached regarding the action which needs to be taken. This will naturally vary, depending on the seriousness of the incident, and will range from working with the family and with the child remaining in the home, to prosecuting the offending adult and placing the child in long-term foster care.

The teacher's involvement with the future planning of the life of a child of school age who is to remain at home is paramount, in view of the need to maintain close supervision of the child's emotional state and school progress.

CHOREA – *see* Cerebral Palsy

CHOREO-ATHETOSIS – *see* Cerebral Palsy

COELIAC DISEASE

Coeliac disease occurs in about 1 in 1000 children. It occurs as a result of an intolerance of the intestines to the protein gliadin, which is found in wheat. When this condition presents in early infancy, the child fails to gain weight and has severe diarrhoea. By the time the child starts school, the diagnosis has usually been made and a special diet already started.

The diet consists of the avoidance of all wheat-containing foods. Mothers of children with coeliac disease are usually familiar with the diet and are able to discuss various items with the school catering services. It is advantageous to arrange a visit to the school from the dietitian who normally supervises the child and the diet can be discussed fully with the staff. Apart from the strict avoidance diet, there is no other restriction in a child with coeliac disease.

CONGENITAL HEART DISEASE – *see*
Heart Murmur

CYSTIC FIBROSIS

Prevalence

Cystic fibrosis or mucoviscidosis is a rare inherited disease which occurs in about 1 in 2000 children.

Presentation

As a result of a probable chemical defect, the mucous-secreting glands in the body secrete very thick and tenacious mucous. In the case of the lungs, this causes them to be blocked and leads to severe and recurrent chest infections and, as a result of this and the ensuing damage, also leads to a considerable degree of breathlessness and limitation of physical activity. The thick mucous secretion also blocks the pancreatic duct and prevents the flow of pancreatic juice into the intestines. This results in a failure to absorb fat which, consequently, accumulates in the stool.

Treatment

The medical treatment consists of daily physiotherapy to encourage chest drainage. Regular participation in games, particularly using the trampoline, is most important.

Children with cystic fibrosis may be required to take regular antibiotics to prevent respiratory infection, or may need them in the form of intermittent courses of treatment. The absence of pancreatic juice necessitates the taking of tablets or capsules containing pancreatic enzymes at the same time as meals or snacks. Additional vitamins and preparations containing a high number of calories are also necessary.

The child's participation in exercise and sport in school should be encouraged and limited only to the extent of the child's own disability. Naturally, each child will differ in this respect.

School Work

Since many children with cystic fibrosis spend considerable periods in hospital for treatment, it is important that they are given every assistance to continue with their school work. Most children's wards have a teacher who visits the hospital on a daily basis and who is able to instruct those of junior school age with their work. Difficulties may arise in children of secondary school age because of the diversity of subjects which they are studying and special arrangements may have to be made. It is helpful if work can be brought into the hospital by the child's form teacher so that the child may keep up with his/her peers. To facilitate this, a programme could be co-ordinated by the form teacher and the hospital teacher on a weekly basis during the child's stay in hospital.

CYSTITIS

Cystitis occurs as a result of a bacterial infection of the bladder. It is one of the most common causes of recurrent abdominal pain and many occur at any age, although it is more common in girls than boys.

A child with cystitis complains of lower abdominal pain, frequent passing of small amounts of urine and a discomfort or burning sensation when urine is passed. Occasionally, there is hesitancy (although the child is desperate to go to the toilet, no urine is passed). This may be as a result of pain, or because of a sensation of the need to urinate in the absence of urine in the bladder. If a teacher observes a child with any of these symptoms, they should report the matter to the parents with an explanation of the possible causes, so that arrangements may be made for the child to be referred for further investigation.

In a child in whom a diagnosis has already been made, it is important that the child empties the bladder whenever the need arises. The less formality that the child has to go through to achieve this, the better. Occasionally, the child may delay emptying the bladder because of being distracted. If this is obvious to the teacher, then the child should be reminded to go to the toilet at regular intervals.

Since recurrence of infection can occur as a result of infrequent emptying of the bladder, prolonged waiting without a break should be avoided (e.g. rehearsing for school concerts, etc.).

Some children will require treatment with regular urinary antiseptics or antibiotics, if they have had severe infections. Others require courses of treatment intermittently. Most of the time, such antibiotics are given at home on a twice daily basis.

DEAFNESS – *see* Hearing Defects

DEPRESSION

Many children experience periods of sadness and mild depression at some stage during their childhood or adolescence. Given an opportunity to discuss their problems and anxieties, with some guidance, they are usually able to understand and resolve their difficulties with a corresponding improvement in their mood.

Transient periods of mild depression may be due to problems with school work, with friends or peers, with home situations, or with future prospects. Problems with school work may arise because of poor progress, difficulty with certain subjects and, in some children, an inability to maintain a standard set by themselves or their parents. Help may be given by additional tuition, reviewing subject choice, or counselling regarding academic progress. Problems with friends and peers occur because of quarrels, teasing, victimisation, or bullying. Quarrels between children (particularly between girlfriend and boyfriend) are common and are usually short-lived. Teasing, victimisation and bullying should not be tolerated as they can lead to school refusal, poor academic progress and further depression and it is important that steps should be taken to identify perpetrators, so that they may be counselled and dealt with. Problems caused by situations in the home may be due to parental marital troubles, divorce, quarrelling, physical or sexual abuse, parental unemployment and family financial worries. Although counselling a child who has problems at home may not solve all the likely difficulties, it is important that the child has an opportunity to discuss such matters with someone not directly involved, so that possible avenues of help may be identified. The uncertainty of job prospects and college or university entrance undoubtedly causes problems in many adolescents and early career advice and planning may be helpful.

Among those children who present in school as being sad and miserable, there are some that can be identified as being truly depressed and these may require a different approach to treatment.

There has been much debate regarding the incidence of true depression during puberty and adolescence and the diagnosis will depend on the criteria which are adopted. It is suggested by some that depression at this age presents in one of two forms, either masked depression or depressive equivalents.

In masked depression, there is no change in mood but there are instead other behavioural manifestations such as hyperactivity, aggression, delinquency and learning difficulties. Depressive equivalents manifest themselves as physical complaints such as headaches, abdominal pain, tiredness and fatigue.

Other authors believe that in order to make a diagnosis of depression, there must be present the primary symptoms of sadness, misery and also some expression of self-depreciation and low self-esteem. In association with this group of symptoms, at least two other secondary symptoms should be present including aggressive behaviour, suicidal thoughts, sleep disturbance, a falling-off of school work and performance, loss of appetite, social withdrawl and physical complaints.

Since sadness and misery are not uncommon amongst children of this age, only extreme variations in mood should be considered abnormal. Some of the secondary symptoms are not specific to depression and are commonly found in disturbed children.

Suspicion of depression in a child should be dealt with by an initial discussion between an educational psychologist, the parents and the teacher. Subsequent referral to a child psychiatrist should be arranged if the symptoms are severe or persistent.

DIABETES

Prevalence

Diabetes occurs in about 1 in every 1000 children but recent evidence suggests that its incidence is increasing slightly.

Presentation

Diabetes in children, or juvenile diabetes, arises as a result of an absence of insulin which is normally produced in the pancreas. The function of insulin is to utilise the carbohydrate content of the diet (potatoes, bread, sugar, etc.). Normally, carbohydrates are absorbed from the intestine into the blood stream in the form of glucose. Insulin is responsible for converting this into energy used by all the cells of the body, particularly muscles. A failure in the production of insulin will, therefore, result in a rise in the level of blood sugar. The consequences of this are that the child becomes increasingly tired, loses weight and develops an excessive thirst accompanied by an increased frequency of urination.

Treatment

Diabetes in childhood requires treatment with insulin given by injection along with a regular, balanced diet – the purpose of both being to maintain a fairly normal blood glucose level. This is controlled by regular testing of the urine or, in some instances, of blood glucose.

Insulin
Insulin is administered by injection usually before breakfast and often before the evening meal as well. It is only rarely that insulin will need to be given during school hours.

Diet
If the child remains at school for the midday meal, it is essential to discuss the diet with the school health services, the parents

and, if possible, with the dietitian from the hospital where the child is being treated. Most paediatric departments undertaking the care of diabetic children will willingly arrange a visit to the school by the dietitian and often by a health visitor or nurse specially assigned to the diabetic clinic, to discuss such matters with the teaching and catering staff. Necessary adjustments to school meals are usually straightforward and at most, only require sbustitution of one food product for another and basic measurements.

Sugar and sweet foods should be avoided, except in emergencies. Any protein-rich foods, such as meat and almost any vegetable, can be eaten normally. Carbohydrate food will need to be given according to the child's diet and needs to be fixed for each meal. A certain amount of carbohydrate will be required mid-morning and mid-afternoon, as a snack.

LOW BLOOD GLUCOSE (HYPOGLYCAEMIA)

One of the most important aspects of caring for a diabetic child at school is the early recognition and treatment of low blood sugar. These episodes are referred to as insulin reactions, hypoglycaemic attacks or, more commonly, in the child's own jargon as 'hypos'.

The blood sugar may become too low as a result of any of the following factors:

1 Giving too much insulin.
2 Having inadequate carbohydrate in the diet.
3 Being late for a meal or snack.
4 Undertaking excessive physical activity.

When a child's blood sugar becomes excessively low, certain symptoms will be noticed. Many of these may have already been experienced during the child's initial stay in hospital. A child may therefore be able to inform the teacher of an impending hypoglycaemic attack. Early recognition may enable the child to rectify the situation quickly but, since confusion is often present as a result of hypoglycaemia, this may not always be possible.

The symptoms of hypoglycaemia are: hunger, shakiness, headache, double vision, occasionally nausea and vomiting and, less frequently, tingling and numbness of the lips and tongue.

However, because the child may not always recognise the symptoms, the diagnosis will often need to be made by the teacher. The teacher will therefore need to recognise different features of the attack and these are:

Early manifestations

– confusion;
– irritability;
– pallor and sweating.

Later manifestations

– listlessness;
– wandering attention;
– naughtiness and stubbornness;
– difficulty in reading;
– difficulty in answering questions;
– unreasonable tearfulness;
– unsteadiness.

If these symptoms are treated promptly, normal behaviour will usually return within five to ten minutes. Failure to treat them will result in the child becoming unconscious.

Treatment of Low Blood Glucose

All diabetic children should carry with them, at all times, either sugar or glucose tablets. Teachers who have a child with diabetes in their class should follow the golden rule, 'if in doubt, give sugar'. If the child or teacher notices the onset of an attack, sugar should be given at once, in the form of either:

– two heaped teaspoonfuls or three sugar lumps in water; or
– a glucose tablet to suck; or
– a boiled sweet to suck.

If there is no improvement after five minutes, the dose of sugar should be repeated. When the child recovers, it may be advisable to give an additional biscuit, a piece of chocolate or a sandwich.

If the child develops a hypoglycaemic attack and becomes unconscious, DO NOT give anything by mouth, in view of the danger of inhalation into the lungs. A doctor should be summoned and, if one is not immediately available, the child should be transferred by ambulance to the nearest hospital.

Prevention of Attacks

Prevention of these attacks is obviously preferable even to early treatment. Children should not miss their mid-morning or mid-afternoon snacks; they should not be late for their midday meal and, above all, they should take extra carbohydrate before strenuous exercise.

In view of the danger of hypoglycaemia, keeping a child behind after normal school hours may not be an ideal form of punishment. It would be more advisable to give the child additional work to carry out at home.

Education

With proper management, the diabetic child can, and should, be educated at an ordinary school. There are, however, some diabetic children who, because of difficulty in controlling their diabetes, social factors, or emotional problems, require special schooling. The diabetic child will benefit from periods spent with other diabetic children at camps organised by the British Diabetic Association. This helps the child realise that others have similar problems and the experience fosters a spirit of self-confidence and independence.

Physical Education

It is important that every effort is made to make the school life of a diabetic child as near normal as possible. Since it is a relatively uncommon condition, the child may be one of only two or so in the school who suffer from it and, understandably, will often feel lonely and different from other members of the class. It is particularly important that the child does not use diabetes as an excuse not to participate in school activities which are disliked. Since physical education is such a vital part of school life, the child should always take part.

Certain strenuous exercise may result in the blood glucose being used up rapidly, with a consequent fall in level causing a 'hypo' attack. This can easily be prevented by giving the child a snack of milk, biscuits, or chocolate before activity takes place. Occasionally, it may be necessary for a child to require snacks during or immediately after any activity.

Special precautions need to be taken with certain activities, especially: swimming, cross country running, and gymnastic work on high appliances. For these activities, a child must be under the supervision of an informed member of the teaching staff.

The diabetic child should not be prohibited from attending school outings. If necessary, picnic meals can be prepared by the parents, which would obviate any dietary problems.

DIARRHOEA AND VOMITING

Diarrhoea and vomiting often occur in children and are usually due to an infection of the intestines, due to either a bacteria or a virus. These infections may be transmitted by direct contact from one child to another or by contamination of food. The symptoms of diarrhoea and vomiting occurring together are given the name gastro-enteritis. They may both (independently) be presenting features of other illnesses in childhood.

The term food poisoning covers accidental poisoning through the contamination of food by bacteria, bacterial toxins or chemicals. This may produce either vomiting by itself or vomiting and diarrhoea.

In view of the infectious nature of many of the illnesses causing diarrhoea and vomiting, and the implications as far as school is concerned, most are notifiable to the Community Physician and Environmental Health Officer who should take steps to control the infection.

Certain groups of individuals pose special risks of spreading infection and these are:

1 Food handlers who touch unwrapped food.
2 Health care, nursery or other staff who have direct contact, or who serve food, to susceptible children (i.e. those children listed in 3 below).
3 Children under the age of five years attending nurseries, playschool or nursery schools.
4 Older children and adults with poor standards of hygiene. Exceptionally, this may include children in infants' schools.

The most common infective organisms which produce outbreaks of diarrhoea and vomiting in schools are shigella, salmonella, staphlococcus and certain viruses. Detailed guidelines for the control of these infections and the consequent action that has to be taken come under the supervision of the Community Physician and Environmental Health Officer in each health district. The precautions and actions which need to be taken vary slightly from one causative factor to the other and briefly, are as follows:

SHIGELLA (BACILLARY DYSENTERY)

Source
Usually from other infected individuals.

Spread
By faecal-oral contact in young children. It spreads quickly in nursery schools and infant schools, especially where there is poor hygiene and poor toilet facilities.

Exclusion from school
Any child or individual from the aforesaid groups, until they are free from diarrhoea and have 3 negative stool cultures (i.e. no bacterial growth) in a period of 3 days. Any household contact of anyone from these groups should also be excluded until there have been 3 negative stool cultures in 3 days.

SALMONELLA

Source
Raw meat and poultry are the main sources of infection. There is often contamination when raw meat is prepared on working surfaces which are also used for the preparation of cooked meats. Occasionally, contamination may occur when cooked meats are stored next to raw meat. Other sources are tinned meat and tinned fish.

Spread
From contaminated food or faecal-oral routes in young children.

Exclusion from school
Any child or individual from the aforesaid groups until free of symptoms.

Prolonged exclusion from school of anyone in these groups who is free from symptoms, even though Salmonella may continue to be cultured from the stools, is rarely necessary. Exclusion from school of individuals who are symptom free and who have positive stool cultures for Salmonella and who are not in the special groups is rarely, if ever, justified.

The policy with respect to infection due to salmonella typhi (typhoid) and salmonella paratyphi B (paratyphoid) are more complex and detailed, particularly with respect to food handlers and persistent carriers of infection.

STAPHLOCOCCUS

The bacteria staphlococcus is a common bacteria found on the skin and in the nose, and is the cause of skin infections such as boils or infected cuts. It produces a chemical toxin which is responsible for the symptoms.

Source
Infective skin lesions, fingers and nose of food handlers.

Spread
From contamination of cooked foods stored at room temperature. Contamination of cream, cream products, cakes and puddings.

Exclusion from school
Any food handler (group 1) found to be the source of infection should be excluded until such time as the lesion has responded to treatment.

VIRUSES

In younger children, many different viruses have been isolated as the causative agents in outbreaks of diarrhoea and vomiting or gastro-enteritis.

Source
Contact with infectious individuals or occasionally by contamination of food.

Spread
Usually by faecal-oral spread.

Exclusion from school
Any individual in the aforesaid groups should be excluded from school until free of symptoms. In one particular infection, that due to a virus called rotavirus, they should not return to school until 7 days after recovery, since the stool may continue to contain the virus up to this length of time.

General Measures

Outbreaks of infection due to these organisms can be prevented or contained by paying particular attention to some basic precautionary measures, as follows:

1 There must be stringent adherence to hygiene measures in kitchens, particularly with respect to the handling and storage of food.
2 Food handlers should report, and be excluded from duties if they have diarrhoea or infected skin lesions.
3 Children or staff who have diarrhoea should seek immediate medical advice and remain home until symptoms have cleared or until advised to return to school.
4 Children should be educated early in life in the importance of personal hygiene.
5 Toilet hygiene of younger children should be supervised.
6 Adequate and hygenic toilet facilities should be maintained in all schools.

DIPLEGIA – *see* Cerebral Palsy

DOWN'S SYNDROME

Down's syndrome is the most common single cause of mental subnormality encountered in the United Kingdom, and is also the commonest condition resulting from an abnormality of the chromosomes. The degree of subnormality varies from child to child, some requiring teaching in schools for severely subnormal or educationally subnormal children whilst others may be educated in ordinary schools.

Prevalence

Down's syndrome occurs in about 1 in every 700 births. Some children have other associated problems which cause early death in infancy and hence, the incidence of Down's in school-children is slightly less.

Cause

Chromosomes are complex protein molecules made up of chains of aminoacids which are found in the nuclei of each cell in the body. When seen under an electron microscope, each chromosome has the appearance of the letter X. There are 46 chromosomes in each cell, 22 of these can be matched into pairs and the remaining two are known as sex chromosomes. In females, they appear like two Xs hence XX and in males, an X and Y, hence XY. Each pair of chromosomes can be identified by their size and are numbered for purposes of recognition from 1 to 22 in gradually decreasing size (1 being the largest pair and 22 the smallest).

The presence of an extra single chromosome or, in some instances, an extra part of a chromosome gives rise to abnormal characteristics in an individual which are peculiar to the chromosome concerned. Likewise, absences of parts of certain chromosomes may also produce characteristic features.

In Down's syndrome, the problems arise as a result of an additional chromosome (trisomy) which is identical in size to the pair numbered 21. Hence, the condition is known also as Trisomy 21.

The risk of having a child with Down's syndrome increases considerably with the age of the mother. However, since child bearing is less common with increasing maternal age, most mothers of children with Down's syndrome are young.

Presentation

Children who have Down's syndrome are usually easy to identify due to their characteristic appearance and the similarity they bear to each other. These characteristics are:

- They are short in stature, have fair, soft hair, a flat rounded head and sloping eyes.
- Their hands are short and square, have a single crease across the palm and often have a little finger which turns inwards.
- Their early development is delayed both intellectually and physically.
- They are generally happy and contented children, but some may demonstrate a degree of obstinacy, particularly during puberty.
- A number have associated congenital heart defects and many have an increased tendency to developing respiratory infections.

Action by Teacher

There is no special generalised measure, each child should be treated according to his/her own individual level of educational potential and behaviour. They should be encouraged to participate in all extra school activities, particularly in sports such as swimming. However, direct body contact sports (in particular rugby) should be avoided. The reason for this is that in many children with Down's syndrome, a small defect has been found in the bones of the spine near to the base of the skull. This may result in a degree of instability which can cause dislocation.

DRUG ABUSE

In today's society, the abuse of drugs has become an increasing problem, and in communities where there is extreme social or emotional deprivation it has reached epidemic proportions. The reason for this increase is multifactorial and relates to the easy availability of most drugs, together with the existence of a sub-culture of drug takers to which adolescents may feel attracted. Adolescents so attracted, often already have emotional problems, low educational attainment, and may be victims of a disrupted family life. Adverse social factors are frequently quoted as being causative; these may include poverty, low economic status of the family, overcrowded areas and areas where there is a relatively high concentration of under-privileged minority groups. The association between these factors and addiction is, however, not specific. Many children experiment with drugs in order to experience their effects and often, may only do so on one or two occasions. The regular user not only runs the high risk of addiction but may, by changing from one group of drugs to another, end up with more toxic and dependent ones.

Presentation

The symptoms of drug abuse vary slightly from one group to another, but there are certain non-specific signs which can be recognised. These are:

1 Behavioural changes with exaggerated mood swings and irritability.
2 Lack of concentration and deterioration in school work, without obvious reason.
3 Unexplained absences from school.
4 Deterioration in health and appearance.
5 Deterioration in attitude to work, discipline and authority.

Drugs can be divided into three main groups: **common**, **less common** and **infrequent**. The **common** drugs are those such as *solvents* (e.g. glue, varnish etc.) and *hallucinogens* (e.g. cannabis, 'magic' mushrooms and LSD). The **less common** drugs are *stimulants* (e.g. amphetamines and cocaine) and *sedatives* (e.g. barbiturates and tranquilisers). The **infrequent** drugs are *opiates* (e.g. morphine and heroin). The effect each group has, and the means of recognising the effects, will be dealt with under specific headings.

SOLVENTS

This is probably the most common form of drug abuse amongst today's youth, although it is not necessarily confined to this particular age group. A variety of solvents is employed although this form of abuse is more commonly refered to as 'glue sniffing'. The solvents used are any which contain the volatile hydrocarbon toluene. Toluene is found in glue, contact adhesives, typing correction fluid, nail varnish, paint thinners and lighter fuel.

The vapours of the solvents are inhaled from a rag, or from a bag held up to the face. Occasionally, a plastic bag is smeared with the substance and the bag held over the head.

Immediate effects
The immediate effects are very similar to those found in alcohol intoxication but come on much more quickly, are shorter lasting and are not followed by a hangover. The remaining effects are:

– confusion and disorientation;
– loss of inhibition and euphoria;
– alteration of perception;
– aggression and mood liability;
– slurred speech;
– unsteadiness.

Later effects:
– drowsiness;
– hallucinations;
– double vision;
– ringing in the ears.

Permanent effects
Persistent solvent abuse may lead to major toxic effects on the kidneys, liver, heart and central nervous system. Its effect on the brain can lead, eventually, to convulsions and coma. At any time during the process of 'sniffing', vomiting and inhalation of vomit can occur with subsequent effects and lack of oxygen. It is estimated that over 60 deaths due to solvent abuse occurred in the United Kingdom between 1971 and 1981.

Signs of abuse
Apart from the obvious signs previously mentioned, such as acute intoxication, there may be some evidence between bouts of 'sniffing' which will assist the teaching staff to identify the problem. The signs may include redness and watering of the eyes, a hacking cough, excessive nasal discharge, spots, redness or red rings around the mouth, stomach pains and sickness, numbness and tingling in the hands and feet and possibly an odour of solvent on the breath or clothes.

Action by Teacher

Teachers should be actively involved with the health staff in a programme of health education with the aim of preventing solvent abuse. In areas where abuse is common, there may be established multidisciplinary groups which can be approached for assistance to deal with a child suspected of 'sniffing'. Often the child itself will approach such a group for help. In certain areas, local education and social work services have produced their own guidelines for teachers.

HALLUCINOGENS

MARIJUANA

Marijuana is obtained from the crushed leaves and flowering tops of *cannabis sativa*, the hemp plant. The flowering tops secrete a resin which, when collected and compressed, is called hashish – it is four to eight times more potent than marijuana. Marijuana, also known as hemp, grass, hash or weed, is smoked by rolling it with tobacco in a home-made cigarette known as a 'joint' or a 'reefer'. Hashish is smoked in a wide variety of small pipes. Both preparations may be ingested with food, although this is uncommon.

Occasional users generally smoke in groups where the ritual of rolling and sharing a 'joint' is an integral part of the social contact. More chronic smokers frequently smoke alone.

Immediate effects

These occur within minutes of inhalation and reach a maximum in about an hour, finally disappearing in about 3 hours. The effects of the drug is naturally dependent on the amount present. The effects are as follows:

Physiological
— rapid heart rate;
— redness of the eyes;
— flushing of the skin;
— dryness of the mouth and throat;
— tremors of the hands;
— unsteadiness;
— nausea and vomiting.

Psychological
The psychological effects will depend not only on the amount used but on the personality of the user and the social setting and company in which the drug is used. The effects are:

— enhanced perception of sound, colours and taste;
— euphoria;
— occasionally anxiety and depression;
— hyper-activity and hilarity;
— fleeting ideas;
— distortion of time and space;
— increased imagination and occasional hallucinations;
— impairment of physical ability and reaction time;
— altered attention span (although attention is maintained in certain situations).

Long-term effects

Long-term effects are usually found in chronic users of marijuana and are as follows:

- increased incidence of bronchitis, sinusitis and throat inflammation;
- depression;
- acute panic reactions and paranoia;
- in certain individuals with psychological problems, an acute psychotic reaction may occur with hallucinations, confusion and depersonalisation.

As with other drug groups, treatment is directed at health education and specialised help for those individuals with associated psychological problems.

'MAGIC' MUSHROOMS

Hallucinogenic mushrooms have been used in parts of South America for many centuries. Their use in this country is becoming more common, particularly in some areas of Wales, where they grow in profusion. The mushroom most commonly used is the liberty cap or *Psilocybe semilanceata*, illustrated examples of which have been published (Watling, 1973). Some children have been known, however, to ingest other mushrooms that have considerably more toxic and serious consequences.

The mushrooms may be eaten raw, dried, or as a stew in boiling water. The effects are due to two toxins, psilocybin and psilocin, which act in a similar way to LSD. The results of ingestion become evident in about 30 minutes and may last up to 6 hours or longer.

Immediate effects
The effects, as with other hallucinogenic drugs, are both physiological and psychological.

Physiological
- rapid pulse rate;
- dilated pupils;
- facial flushing;
- abdominal pain and vomiting.

Psychological
The following visual hallucinations may be experienced:

- flashing coloured lights;

- increased visual perception with colours appearing vivid;
- faces appearing coloured and distorted.

Auditory hallucinations may include hearing voices. Accompanying these, may be a sensation of changes in size of bodily parts, including the tongue; confusion and disorientation; agitation and fright; and a feeling of pins and needles in both hands and feet.

Later effects

The immediate effects have usually disappeared in about 6 hours but some of the psychological effects may last much longer and there have been reports of prolonged psychiatric states occurring which required hospital admission.

One specific problem which may arise, concerns the ingestion of poisonous varieties of mushrooms, the commonest of these being of the genus *Amanita*, which is blamed for most cases of mushroom poisoning and fatalities. Following the ingestion of this variety, there may be some transient effects. There is often a latent period of about 12 hours before severe diarrhoea, abdominal pain and vomiting occurs. This may continue for about 2 to 3 days, after which there is evidence of liver damage, with increasing yellowness of the skin and jaundice. In view of this danger, it is essential that any child admitting to having ingested 'magic' mushrooms should be referred immediately for a medical opinion.

LSD

Lysergic acid diethylamide, or acid, is a less commonly used drug amongst the school population. It is less easily available and its use is usually confined to occasional experiences or 'trips' in the company of other users. Rarely, is it used by individuals on a more regular basis to produce almost constant intoxication; these are the so-called 'acid heads'.

It is available in a variety of forms including impregnated paper, sugar cubes, capsules, or tablets. It may often be mixed with other psychedelic drugs.

The effects of the drug occur within about 20 minutes of ingestion and last up to 12 hours, although fatigue and tension may follow for a further 24 hours.

Immediate effects
The effects are physiological and psychological.

Physiological

- rapid heart rate;
- flushing of face;
- dilated pupils;
- increased alertness
- occasional nausea and vomiting.

Psychological
These effects become evident in about 2 hours and vary between individuals depending on their psychological make-up and mood, and the dose used. The effects are:

- heightened perception;
- sense of unusual clarity;
- apparent slow passage of time;
- body distortion commonly perceived;
- euphoria and excitation;
- depression and panic.

An acute panic reaction is the most common complication with the use of LSD, (the so-called 'bad trip' or 'freak out'). These vary in intensity but have led to suicidal attempts.

Later effects
Adverse reactions are more commonly seen in individuals who are emotionally disturbed even before embarking on experiments with LSD. These include paranoia, depression and 'flash-back' phenomena. In the latter, there occurs the same experience as is found whilst taking the drug, even though the individual has not used the drug for some time.

STIMULANTS

The drugs in this group, which are subject to abuse include:

- amphetamine ('amphets' or 'uppers');
- methyl amphetamine ('speed', 'crystal' or 'meth');
- cocaine ('coke').

AMPHETAMINE GROUP

Amphetamine, Dexedrine or benzadrine ('bennies').

Effects

In low doses, these drugs have the property of increasing alertness, inhibiting sleep and decreasing appetite. It is their mood-elevating properties that make them popular among drug users.

Although the drugs are commonly used orally, they may also be sniffed (as in the case of cocaine) or taken intravenously. The effects are:

– sense of increased activity;
– increased talking;
– feeling of power and intensity.

This is followed by an unpleasant sensation of fatigue and depression ('crashing').

COCAINE

The use of cocaine seems to be confined to the more affluent areas, since it is only available illicitly and it is more expensive than either amphetamine or heroin, and its effects do not last as long.

Immediate effects

– elevation of mood;
– decreased need for food and sleep;
– hyperactivity.

Long-term effects

Frequent 'sniffing' results in irritation of the nose. The individual feels constantly fatigued and depressed and has a sensation of something crawling under the skin (cocaine bug) which causes constant scratching.

SEDATIVES

The most frequently abused drugs in this group are barbiturates, particularly those which have a short-lived effect. Other drugs used in this group are tranquillisers such as Valium and

Librium. Most drugs in this group are available fairly easily and are found in many ordinary households having been obtained from physicians' prescriptions. The drugs are taken by ingestion; they are rarely taken intravenously.

Immediate effects

- sense of tranquillity;
- blunting of inhibitions and anxiety;
- aggression;
- occasionally violent and anti-social behaviour.

Long-term effects

Although the initial effects of sedatives may be very similar to the early stages of intoxication from alcohol, the hypnotic effect of this group of drugs eventually becomes evident. This results in drowsiness, depression, impairment of judgment and performance and, occasionally, hyper-excitability. These after-effects can persist for many hours after drug taking and will depend on the type of drug used and the tolerance of the individual.

OPIATES

Morphine and heroin are extractions of the poppy plant, *Papaver somniferum*. It is, fortunately, a rarely used drug among adolescents attending school. Because many who have acquired an addiction will have already identified with a similar peer group out of school, they will be regular truants or early 'drop-outs'.

The heroin generally available on the street ('smack', 'junk' or 'dope') is initially used by sniffing. In order to maintain the initial effects, users begin to inject it into the skin ('skin poppers') and finally, intravenously ('main-lining').

Immediate effects

- a sense of relaxation and peace;
- euphoria;
- relief of worry and tension.

When given intravenously, there is a warm feeling or 'rush' immediately after the injection.

Long-term effects

As the individual's tolerance to heroin increases, the euphoric effects diminish and are replaced by a physical dependency. There are many complications which arise secondary to its use, from infection at the sites of injection to hepatitis, lung infections, pneumonia and nervous system disorders. Recent evidence seems to suggest that the street price for heroin may be falling, with the possibility that its use may increase as it did in the 1970s. It has been estimated that heroin addiction was the major cause of death in males between the ages of fifteen to thirty-five in New York in 1971.

DYSKINESIA – *see* Cerebral Palsy

DYSLEXIA

Dyslexia usually manifests itself at the age of seven or eight years, when it becomes obvious that a child is having difficulty in reading. This is accompanied by difficulty in writing and spelling and often by reversal of letters or words. There is often a family history of reading problems.

A useful check list for a diagnosis of dyslexia has been formulated by Miles (1974), which is applicable to children of eight-and-a-half years and under. The relevant questions are:

1 Is the child having particular difficulty with reading?
2 Is the child having particular difficulty spelling?
3 Does this surprise the parent?
4 Does the child seem normal in areas unrelated to spelling and reading?
5 Does the child reverse figures (e.g. 15 for 51 and 6 for 9)?
6 Does the child reverse letters (e.g. p for q and d for b)?
7 Does the child make numerical calculations using blocks, fingers or marks on paper?
8 Does the child have unusual difficulties remembering numerical tables?
9 Was the child late developing social speech?
10 Is the child unusually clumsy?

According to Miles, three or four positive responses indicate that the child requires full psychological assessment and further discussion regarding possible placement or special remedial teaching.

DYSMENORRHOEA

Dysmenorrhoea may be defined as abdominal pain which comes on at a time of a girl's period and which is sufficiently severe to interfere with the normal day-to-day activity of the individual.

At the onset of menstruation (menarche) the early cycles are irregular and frequently no ovum is produced (anovular). This anovular menstruation seldom causes pain and, therefore, the first few periods are usually pain free.

Dysmenorrhoea is more common when mensturation is established. If pain occurs during the first few periods it usually reflects the attitude the girl and her parents have towards menstruation. A simple explanation of the physiology of menstruation may often help.

Treatment

Treatment depends on the amount of pain present and the degree of disability accompanying it. If at all possible, exercise should be encouraged and the girl should join in games or physical education whenever she can. If this is not possible, rest with local warmth applied, such as a hot water bottle, and the use of Aspirin or Codeine will often help.

In persistent and severe cases, ovulation may have to be inhibited by the use of cyclical hormone therapy.

ECZEMA

Eczema is the most common skin condition seen in infancy and childhood. Most infants who suffer from eczema have very few, or no problems by the time they reach school age and about 50% of schoolchildren cease to have problems by the time they are thirteen.

Cause

Various factors probably contribute to the cause of eczema but the mechanism by which the characteristic skin changes are produced is not clearly understood.

Many children with eczema also have hay fever and asthma and although there is no simple relationship between eczema and allergy, there is little doubt that allergy plays an important part. However it is difficult to explain the presence of very dry skin and a low itch threshold which children with eczema have on an allergic basis alone.

Presentation

The skin in eczema is very dry, flaky and intensely itchy. Major areas of inflammation are found on the insides of the elbows, wrists, behind the knees, on the ankles, around the ears and around the eyes. The itching causes the child to scratch so furiously that areas of the skin break and start to bleed. In addition, the constant scratching worsens the primary condition and may allow secondary infection in some lesions.

Since eczema is only due to an individual's abnormal response to constitutional or other factors, it is important to realise that it is not catching and therefore, a child with eczema presents no danger to any other person in the class.

Treatment

1 In some children, certain materials are found to cause irritation such as wool or synthetic fibre. However, cotton is usually well tolerated.

2 Most children with eczema should avoid washing with soap and soap substitutes can be made available at school.

3 Occasionally, it may be necessary for some of the younger children to wear gloves so as to reduce damage to their own skin than can be caused by scratching.

4 In some children, dietary restriction of certain foods has been beneficial. Such a programme of dietary control, however, needs to be carefully supervised by a dietitian.

5 Antihistamines are given orally to reduce the itchiness. These may be Vallergan, Phenergan or Piriton. Occasionally, it may be necessary to give them at school although, in general, they are usually prescribed for use at night.

6 Numerous preparations of oils, bath and skin emolients, creams and ointments are used by children with eczema. These vary depending on the severity of the eczema, the response of the individual child and the preference of the skin specialist supervising their treatment.

There are no specific restrictions to a child's activity at school if he or she has eczema.

See also   Allergy

ENTERITIS – *see* Diarrhoea and Vomiting

EPILEPSY

'Epilepsy is the only common disorder I know where the sufferer is more handicapped by the attitude of society than by his own disability' (Lennox, 1960).

Prevalence

In the age group of five to fourteen years, the incidence of epilepsy is 8 in 1000. About 2 in 1000 will have developed epilepsy secondary to another primary disease and will require special education. Thus the prevalence in a normal school is 6 per 1000.

Presentation

Epilepsy can present in a variety of different forms but the commoner types fall into three main categories which are as follows:

GRAND MAL (MAJOR) EPILEPSY

In this type of epilepsy, there occurs what is commonly termed an 'epileptic fit'. The child is seen to stiffen suddenly and fall to the floor. This event may be preceeded by a vocal sound or, on occasions, by a period of irritability or abnormal behaviour. During this initial phase (the 'tonic phase') the breath is held, the teeth and hands are tightly clenched and the child's face becomes blue.

Immediately following this, there are jerking movements of the arms and legs and, occasionally, of the whole body. Associated with this (the 'clonic phase') there may be gnashing movements of the jaw, upward rolling movement of the eyes, frothing at the mouth and, at times, incontinence of urine.

When the jerking movements have ended, the child becomes quite limp and relaxed and may recover quickly. If the attack is prolonged, it may be followed by a deep sleep, at the end of which the child may be irritable, tired and may complain of a headache.

PETIT MAL (MINOR) EPILEPSY

In this type of epilepsy, the child appears periodically to have episodes of staring, associated with an unawareness of what is happening in the surrounding environment. Attacks last a few seconds at a time and may occur as often as twenty times a day. If episodes occur whilst a child is handling objects, the grip may suddenly be relaxed and the object fall to the floor. Such children are frequently thought to be clumsy and are often accused of day-dreaming or of lacking concentration. If the attacks occur frequently, the child may lose the continuity of the lesson, with subsequent deterioration in school progress.

Petit mal is more common in girls than boys and reaches a peak at the age of nine. Attacks can be precipitated by over-breathing or by flashing lights. Probably, the first indication of petit mal is a gradual deterioration of school work. This deterioration may also occur in a child who is already on treatment but, because of poor compliance or inadequate control, is having an increased number of attacks.

TEMPORAL LOBE EPILEPSY

Attacks of temporal lobe epilepsy may manifest themselves in a variety of different ways. Occasionally there is no attack as such, save that the child experiences an odd sensation, some-times terrifying, and usually impossible to describe.

An attack may result in a sensation of a change in body image or size – for example, shrinking of the whole or part of the body, the so called 'Alice in Wonderland' effect. This may, at times, be reflected as apparent in other individuals' body shape or size. The attacks may take the form of short episodes of tongue protrusion or lip smacking, accompanied by grimac-ing. On rare occasions the child may be unable to speak, despite being fully conscious. There may sometimes be periods of aggression and difficult behaviour associated with rather purposeless, repetitive movements of the arms.

What to do for an Attack

In the case of petit mal and temporal lobe epilepsy, the attacks are usually short and the child rarely falls to the floor. The following remarks, therefore, refer mainly to grand mal epilepsy:

1   The child should be left where he/she falls, but any objects, such as a desk or chair, should be moved away to reduce the risk of injury.
2   Tight clothing around the neck or upper chest should be loosened.
3   The child should be turned to lie on one side in the 'recovery' position.
4   The child should remain in this position until recovery has occurred.
5   DO NOT insert hard objects between the child's teeth to prevent tongue biting. This is rare in children but, if it does occur, a folded leather belt could be used.
6   DO NOT use excessive restraint.

Treatment

Various drugs are used in the treatment of epilepsy. There are four main reasons for this:

1   Different types of epilepsy require different drugs.
2   Children do not always respond to the same drug.
3   Doctors have individual drug preferences.
4   Some children have side effects to some drugs but not to others.

In order to maintain adequate levels of the drug in the blood stream, it may be necessary for tablets or medication to be administered during school time. The drugs that are commonly used in the treatment of epilepsy are these:

Grand mal epilepsy – Epanutin (Phenytoin), Phenobarbitone, Epilim (Sodium Valproate), Tegretol (Carbemazapine).
Petit mal – Zarontin (Ethosuximide), Epilim.
Temporal lobe epilepsy – Tegretol.

Side effects of drugs
The most important side effects to observe and report during school hours are tiredness, sleepiness, lack of concentration, irritability, hyperactivity and behavioural changes.

Education

Educational attainment will vary according to the severity of the epilepsy and, in particular, with the age of onset. Epilepsy starting in infancy carries a poorer outlook for intellectual ability than when it starts in later childhood. In a study carried out in Scotland in 1977, a total of 285 children with epilepsy, attending normal school, were tested for their reasoning ability. When the results were compared to a group of normal children matched for age, it was found that the boys tested had a lower score but the girls' score was the same.

It is completely unfounded that children with epilepsy are more likely to have a fit when they are angered, aggravated or opposed.

Physical Activity

Children with epilepsy should lead as normal a school life as possible. One must, however, consider which activities should be allowed and which should be prohibited. It should be stressed that attacks are less likely to occur when children are active and involved than when they are bored. The most usual activities are swimming, sports and physical education.

Swimming
Although the risk of drowning is very low, it is thought to be about four times as likely as in children without epilepsy. However, if a child is supervised by an informed life-guard or swimming companion, he/she can swim in safety.

All schools should adopt the 'pairing' system whereby children are advised to swim in pairs. This provides additional safety for children with epilepsy as well as for children who are weak swimmers. This would not obviate the need for life-guard surveillance. However, the following swimming activities should be prohibited:

- swimming under water;
- diving into deep water;
- swimming in lakes, rivers or the sea, even with a life-guard;
- horseplay.

If the child is known to have frequent attacks, swimming should be limited to short periods and then allowed only with individual supervision. It is believed by some observers that competitive swimming is not advisable in view of the fact that the degree of stress and exhaustion could precipitate an attack. This will depend not only on the severity of the child's epilepsy, but also on the child's physical condition and fitness.

Sport
As with any activity, there should be a balance between the child's need to compete and participate and the limitation which his/her condition imposes. It is probably better to channel the child's interest into sports such as tennis, cricket and athletics. Direct body contact sports, particularly those with an increased risk of head injury, should be avoided, and boxing, judo, karate and wrestling should be prohibited.

Other physical education
Participation in a normal physical education programme should be encouraged, apart from rope climbing, climbing on wall bars, parallel bars and trampoline work.

EYESIGHT – *see* Visual Defects

FOOD POISONING – *see* Diarrhoea and Vomiting

GERMAN MEASLES (RUBELLA)

German measles is characterised by the presence of a fine, red rash, the onset and progression of which is very rapid. There are very few, if any, constitutional symptoms.

Transmission

By droplet or direct contact with an infected child, or by articles freshly contaminated by nasal secretion of such a child.

Incubation Period

From 14 to 21 days; average 16 to 18 days.

Infectious Period

From 7 days before, to approximately 5 days after the appearance of the rash.

A teacher who is in the early stages of pregnancy (up to 2 months) who has direct contact with a child with German measles, particularly if she has not been immunised against German measles, or has not had the infection, should arrange to be seen by her family doctor or obstetrician for tests of susceptibility to the infection to be carried out.

GLANDULAR FEVER
(INFECTIOUS MONONUCLEOSIS)

The presentation in this condition varies from a mild flu-like illness to a more severe situation with tonsillitis, swollen lymph glands in the neck, groins and elsewhere, swelling of the spleen, hepatitis, a rash and extreme listlessness.

Transmission

Probably by droplets from the nose and throat, by saliva or by kissing.

Incubation Period

Probably from 2 to 6 weeks.

Infectious Period

Unknown – probably only during the acute illness.

GLUE SNIFFING – *see* Drug Abuse

HAEMOPHILIA

Haemophilia occurs as a result of a defect in one of the factors necessary for successful blood clotting. It is a genetically-transmitted disease which affects males almost exclusively. Thirteen factors present in the blood are necessary to produce clotting; the factor absent in haemophilia is known as anti-haemophilic globulin (AHG), or Factor VIII.

The result of the absence of AHG is that the time taken for the blood to clot is longer than normal. This, in turn, may cause extensive haemorrhage or bruising following minimal trauma. The bruising may be superficial or deeper into a muscle, or at times there may be haemorrhage into a joint.

Treatment

The treatment of severe bruising or bleeding into a joint is by the intravenous administration of Factor VIII. This is usually given at a centre specialising in the care of haemophilia, but some boys have their own supply of Factor VIII which they administer themselves at home. Factor VIII is prepared from blood donated at transfusion centres, and in the UK it is now heat treated to eliminate the risk of any viral transmission. Prior to this method of treatment, some batches of Factor VIII and a related blood clotting agent, Factor IX, were infected with the virus which is responsible for AIDS.

The majority of the 700 children in this country known to have haemophilia have been tested for the antibody to this virus, known as the human immudodefficiency virus (HIV). Some 35% have been found to have positive antibodies and are carriers of the virus. As these children gradually attain school-leaving age, there will be a corresponding reduction in the number remaining who are HIV positive. To date, it is expected that only a small proportion of those will develop AIDS. (In the USA, about 10% of those with HIV antibodies have developed AIDS and it is thought that the percentage of HIV-positive haemophiliac patients who develop AIDS will be even less.)

Physical Education

In view of the high risk of bruising due to trauma, direct contact sports such as rugby, soccer, boxing, judo, etc., should be avoided. As an alternative, it is preferable to channel the boy's interests into sports such as swimming or tennis.

There should be no restriction in any other aspect of school life except that arrangements may have to be made if the child is to be away for a few days with a group from school. If this is the case it is necessary to ascertain the nearest haemophilia centre (address from Haemophilia Society) or alternatively, facilities should be available for the transportation and storage of the child's own Factor VIII in case it needs to be given.

HEAD LICE

Head lice are small, flat-backed insects about 1–2 mm in length. They are greyish/white in colour and live amongst the hair of the scalp. They feed off scalp blood and have a life expectancy of about 30 days, 2 days if they are away from the head. During their lifetime, each lays about 300 eggs.

Prevalence

In the late 1970s and early 1980s there was an upsurge in the incidence of head lice among school children. The incidence has been falling gradually since the beginning of the century, with a temporary increase only during the two World Wars and during a period in the 1960s when the lice developed resistence to the treatment then available.

The reason for the most recent increase cannot be explained, but it is not due to any return of resistence to treatment since the agents used continue to be effective. The most common age of infestation is between four and six years and it may be that, with the less formal classroom arrangements, there is closer contact between children and hence, easier transfer of head lice from head to head (head lice cannot jump or hop). Another possible explanation is the change in hair styles and in grooming. Frequent combing or brushing of the hair kills a proportion of the lice present. Hair length has little effect, although, if anything, lice prefer short hair.

Presentation

1   The child who is infected constantly scratches the scalp. The itching produced by the head lice is an allergic reaction to the injection of its saliva into the skin. The first few thousand bites cause no reaction, leave no mark and pass unnoticed. Once the child has been sensitised, however, further bites become very itchy. Fifty lice will produce about 200 bites every day.

2   Since the reaction to the bite is an allergic one, there may often be generalised symptoms (e.g. the child may feel tired, listless and restless) – hence the expression, 'feeling lousy'.

3   Observation of the lice may be difficult as they move very swiftly, but if the hair is parted quickly, they may be seen amongst the roots.

4   The most consistent observable finding is the presence of eggs. Live eggs are flesh coloured and are found towards the base of the hair to which they are attached. Hatched eggs or nits appear white and are found further along the length of the hair. They in themselves are of no significance, but are an indication of the length of infestation. Since hair grows about 1 cm a month, a hatched egg found 6 cm from the root indicates that the infestation has been present for 6 months.

Occasionally, medical conditions of the scalp can give rise to small white bodies similar to nits to the naked eye, but which can be distinguished with a hand lens. Nits are rounded bodies attached to the side of a hair.

Treatment

The agents used are: Carbaryl, Malathion and Lindane. These are available as lotions or shampoos. Usually, the treatment is repeated during a period of up to 7 days.

Exclusion from school is usually unnecessary as by the time lice have been detected, the infestation may have been present for 4 to 6 months.

HEADACHE – *see* Migraine

HEARING DEFECTS

Presentation

A child who has poor hearing may present with a variety of different problems in school other than merely complaining of poor hearing. These manifestations may be as follows:

1 Poor school progress.
2 Slow or no response to commands and questions.
3 Mispronunciation of words which may be particularly noticeable when repeating new words.
4 Delay in language development.
5 Inattentiveness or occasional day-dreaming.

Causes

Defective hearing can result from a variety of causes ranging from congenital problems with complete deafness to low grade ear infections with intermittent deafness. There are two main types of deafness:

CONDUCTIVE DEAFNESS

In conductive deafness, there is a failure of conduction of sound waves from the ear drum through the middle ear. It is more common is pre-school children and is usually due to a chronic infection of the middle ear (chronic otitis media) or disease of the ear drum. The deafness fluctuates in intensity, often giving the impression that the child is not paying attention on some days.

SENSORI-NEURAL DEAFNESS

In sensori-neural deafness, there is a failure of transmission of sound from the middle ear via the sensory organ (the cochlea) to the auditory nerve. Transmission failure along the auditory nerve, or a disorder of the part of the brain which receives sound signals, are less common causes of the same type of deafness. The deafness which occurs may fluctuate in intensity but is a permanent disability. Sensori-neural deafness is usually detected in early infancy, either by using hearing screening or because the child is noted not to be responding to normal sounds.

Conductive deafness may not, on the other hand, become obvious until the child is older and, depending on the severity, may go unnoticed for some time. Screening for deafness in schools will be effective in discovering the majority of children with conductive deafness, but some may present signs which would be obvious to the teacher before screening has been undertaken.

Action by the Teacher

A child who is suspected of having poor hearing should be referred via the school health service for detailed hearing tests at an audiology clinic. If the hearing is found to be defective, further referral will be necessary, as a matter of urgency, to the ear, nose and throat specialist. This is because many children who present with conductive deafness require drainage of fluid from the middle ear as a result of chronic infection. This is commonly known as 'glue ear'.

Until such time as arrangements can be made for treatment, the child should sit in the front of the class. If there appears to be a difference in hearing between both ears, the child should sit in a position where the good ear is towards the teacher. The teacher should avoid using loud tones and exaggerated lip movements when talking to a child with a hearing defect. Instead, the teacher should face the child and speak slowly and precisely.

The teacher should remember that a child with a hearing problem may have a fluctuating attention span for school work due to the concentration necessary to be able to hear clearly. It would be helpful to talk to the child's speech therapist to obtain some guidelines on the ideal method of communication and assistance in the classroom.

Established Deafness

A profoundly deaf child may require special placement, either in a partial-hearing unit within an ordinary school or in a school for the deaf. Many other children with hearing loss who require hearing aids may be educated in ordinary schools.

Special Problems

Occasionally, deaf children tend to become withdrawn, frustrated and silent. They may have persisting learning difficulties as a result of an inability to discriminate competing or distorted speech. A deaf child may refuse to wear a hearing aid at school. This may be because the aid is faulty and there may be some 'whistling' due to feedback of sounds. It is important to indicate such reluctance to the parents since a faulty aid, ear piece or problems in the ear canal (all of which are possible causes) need to be rectified immediately.

Sign Language

This is used in some special units, but more particularly in schools for the deaf. The Paget Gorman system, which is different from the standard sign language, is used as an adjunct to speech in children with normal hearing who are suffering from a communication disorder.

See also   Cerebral Palsy

HEART DEFECTS

The majority of heart problems encountered during childhood are due to congenital abnormalities in the development of the heart. There may be narrowing of one of the major blood vessels or of a heart valve, a defect in the walls between the chambers, or a persistence of a channel of communication which should have closed after birth.

Many of these problems will have been corrected surgically before the child starts school; some will be correct later, and the remainder may not require correction or may not be amenable to surgery.

The limitation which will need to be put on a child with a heart defect will be dependent on the type of lesion and the severity. It is therefore essential that each child is discussed with the school doctor, health visitor, or paediatrician supervising his/her care in order to agree an acceptable programme of activity. Many children may be allowed to participate in normal physical activity. Others may be allowed to do all physical activity except competitive sport. Some, because of the degree of associated breathlessness and tiredness, may have to be excluded from any active physical exercise. In the latter group, it is important to introduce them to alternative sport, albeit of a less active nature (e.g. indoor bowls, bowling, skittles, table curling etc.).

HEART MURMURS

When one listens to the heart with a stethoscope, there are two distinct sounds to be heard over each of the four valves. A murmur is a softer sound which is heard in some children and it occurs between the two heart sounds. Every child with congenital heart disease has a heart murmur, but the presence of a heart murmur as such does not necessarily indicate that there is any underlying heart problem. Many school children have what is commonly termed an 'innocent murmur', though the heart is normal. These murmurs may be due to the sound made by the flow of blood through blood vessels entering or leaving the heart, through eddies or currents around the valves, or as a result of minor structural defects in the heart itself.

A child who has an innocent murmur should be discussed with the school doctor or paediatrician but, generally speaking, there should be no restriction of physical activity.

HEMIPLEGIA – *see* Cerebral Palsy

HEPATITIS, INFECTIOUS (YELLOW JAUNDICE)

The characteristic feature of infectious hepatitis is the development of jaundice, or a yellowish discolouration of the skin and, particularly, the whites of the eyes. The jaundice is accompanied or occasionally preceeded by nausea, vomiting, abdominal pain and listlessness.

Transmission

This is mainly through the intestine or oral route, and by secretions of the nose and throat.

Incubation Period

From 15 to 50 days; average 25 days.

Infectious Period

The virus has been detected in the blood and faeces 2 to 3 weeks before the onset of jaundice and may still be excreted in the faeces for a period of 3 weeks afterwards. A child with infectious hepatitis should be expected to be away from school for up to 4 weeks.

HYPERACTIVITY

Some children in their early school years exhibit extreme hyperactivity. They have a diminished attention span, are easily distracted and behave impulsively. They are frequently disruptive and have marked mood swings. Their behaviour not only inhibits their own learning process but also, in great part, that of their fellow pupils.

Hyperactivity may be associated with other neurological problems such as cerebral palsy, epilepsy, or mental retardation. It is also occasionally seen in deaf children; hence it is essential to carry out a hearing assessment on every hyperactive child. Other causes include emotional deprivation and inconsistent management in the home. However, most children claimed to be hyperactive are, in fact, not so.

There is often no associated problem, although recent reports have favoured the view that many hyperactive children respond adversely to certain food additives. These are mainly dyes, artificial colourings and flavourings, and spices, which are found in large numbers of commercially available foods.

The child's hyperactive behaviour should be brought to the parents' attention with the suggestion that, in the first instance, it should be discussed with the family doctor and possibly a paediatrician. The educational psychologist should be asked to assess the child's intellectual capabilities, to rule out the possibility of a major underlying cause. Unfortunately, assessment can often be extremely difficult because of the child's poor attention span and distractability when formally tested.

Occasionally, it may be necessary to remove the child to a smaller class where firm, individual attention may help alleviate the situation. In severe cases, special educational placement in either a remedial class or an observation unit may be necessary.

See also   Cerebral Palsy, Child Abuse, Depression, Drug Abuse, Epilepsy

HYPOGLYCAEMIA – *see* Diabetes

JAUNDICE – *see* Hepatitis, Sickle Cell Disease

LEUKAEMIA (ACUTE)

Acute leukaemia is a rare, malignant blood disorder which is caused by the excessive production of abnormal white cells. These cells invade the lymphatic tissue and bone marrow and interfere with normal cell function. The body's normal defence against infection becomes inadequate, as does the mechanism for the formation of red cells and platelets.

The child presents with an increased incidence of infection, pallor, listlessness, bruising and severe nose bleeds.

Treatment

Children with acute leukaemia need to spend long periods in hospital for intensive treatment. The drugs which are employed are extremely toxic and as they suppress normal as well as abnormal white cells, the child's susceptibility to overwhelming infection, even to common ailments such as measles or chicken pox, is considerably higher.

During the period of in-patient treatment, most children are cared for in paediatric units which have a teacher in attendance. Following the child's discharge home and before their return to school, home tuition should be arranged. When the illness is in remission, the child may resume attending school normally.

MEASLES

Measles presents with a fever for about 3 to 4 days prior to the appearance of a widespread, confluent red rash which is worse on the face. The rash is accompanied by red runny eyes, a runny nose and a cough.

Transmission

Usually by direct contact with droplets (e.g. cough) from an infected child. Less commonly, transmission may be airborne, or by indirect contact from articles freshly contaminated by respiratory tract secretions of an infected child.

Incubation Period

From 10 to 12 days.

Infectious Period

From the fifth day of the incubation period to the first few days of the rash appearing.

MENINGITIS

Acute meningitis occurs as the result of infection and inflammation of the meninges or lining of the brain and spinal cord. The infection can be caused by a variety of different bacteria or viruses. Not all cases of meningitis are infectious, and the same organism in one child may produce few or no symptoms, whereas in another child it may produce meningitis. For example, the virus of mumps, which produces inflammation and swelling of the salivary glands in the majority of children may, in some cases, cause meningitis. The most infectious form of meningitis is that due to the bacteria meningococcus.

The main features of meningitis which, in some instances, may appear very rapidly, are fever, headache and vomiting.

Transmission

Probably by direct contact or inhalation of infected droplets. The meningococcus may be found in the upper respiratory tract of children who have no symptoms – that is the child is a healthy carrier.

Incubation Period

This is variable, depending on the organism responsible, but is usally about 1 to 7 days.

Infectious Period

No longer than 24 hours after the beginning of effective treatment.

In the case of meningitis due to the bacteria meningococcus (meningococcal meningitis), it is advisable that all close contacts of the child receive appropriate preventive oral antibiotic therapy. As soon as the presence of this particular organism has been confirmed, which is usually within the first 24 hours of the child's admission to hospital, the community health department is informed and makes the necessary arrangements for the treatment of contacts.

Preventive treatment for meningitis due to any other organism is unnecessary.

See also   Sickle Cell Disease

MIGRAINE

Recurrent headaches in young children are not as common as abdominal pain but the incidence increases as the child gets older. The most troublesome type of headache encountered is that due to migraine.

Prevalence

Migraine occurs in about 1.4% of children up to the age of seven years and in 4% from the ages of seven to fourteen years.

Presentation

Classically, migraine presents as a one-sided headache. It is often preceeded by visual manifestations which take the form of zig-zag rainbow-coloured lines, moving coloured images, or complete or partial inability to see through one eye. It can be accompanied by nausea and vomiting.

Causes

Migraine is probably due to a variety of causes – for example, stress, food allergy, fatigue, a family history of migraine, or a combination of these.

Children who suffer from migraine are not more intelligent than others, but they do tend to be overly anxious and conscientious regarding their school work. Emotional stress or impending examinations may precipitate an attack.

Increasing attention has been paid to the role of certain foods as precipitating factors in migraine. Agents which are known to be causative include chocolate, coffee, bacon, strong cheese and highly flavoured potato crisps. If any known food is thought to cause migraine, it should be avoided. Loss of sleep and late nights which produce fatigue in a child add to other factors which may be present as precipitating causes.

About 80% of migraine sufferers have a positive family history in one or other parent.

Treatment

Preventive
Certain foods should be avoided if known to be causative agents. The use of preventive drug treatment such as Clonidine (Dixarit) or Pizotifen (Sanomigran) is occasionally necessary if the attacks occur frequently or are severe.

Symptomatic
Normally, analgesic agents such as aspirin or codeine are effective in children with migraine. Some preparations contain either aspirin or paracetamol, together with an agent that prevents vomiting. These are Migravess and Paramax. These are useful if nausea and vomiting are a common accompaniment of the headache. A more specific agent is Ergotamine tartrate, either by itself or in combination with another, such as caffeine (Cafergot or Migril). Ergotamine tartrate may be given by oral spray so that its absorption is not affected by vomiting.

Treatment of Acute Attack

1 The child should be layed down in a quiet, darkened room.
2 If the child takes any specific treatment, this should be administered as early as possible during the attack (e.g. when visual disturbance has started). The earlier treatment commences, the more likely it is to succeed.
3 If vomiting is severe, the parents should be contacted to take the child home or, if in a residential school, the school doctor should be called.

SIMPLE HEADACHES

These are less severe than migraine and may subside if the child's attention is distracted. They occur intermittently in some children, but do not have any of the associated symptoms found in migraine.

MINIMAL BRAIN DYSFUNCTION – *see* Attention Deficit Disorder

MONONUCLEOSIS, INFECTIOUS – *see* Glandular Fever

MUCOVISCIDOSIS – *see* Cystic Fibrosis

MUMPS

Mumps is characterised by the enlargement of the parotid glands which overlie the angles of the jaws. The child may complain of some discomfort in this area, prior to the swelling being obvious. The illness is associated with a high temperature, headache and listlessness.

Transmission

Direct contact or by droplet spread from an infected child, or indirect contact with freshly contaminated articles.

Incubation Period

From 14 to 21 days; average 18 days.

Infectious Period

This is greatest from a few days before the onset of symptoms up to 7 days after parotid swelling is evident. About 30% of children who develop mumps have an inapparent infection.

MUSCULAR DYSTROPHY

This is a rare, progressive, muscular disease which occurs in boys. The incidence is about 1 in 3500. The condition starts with muscle weakness when the child is about three years of age and gradually, between then and the teenage period, there is progressive weakness until such time as the child is confined to a wheelchair. Normal school is possible in the initial stages of the illness, but later special schooling and home tuition will be necessary.

PLANTAR WARTS – *see* Verrucas

RUBELLA – *see* German Measles

SCABIES

Infestation with scabies is due to the mite sarcoptes scabiei which is about 0.3 mm in length. The pregnant female mite burrows into the skin and, over a period of a few weeks, lays a small number of eggs each day in her burrow. The larvae, which hatch from the eggs, emerge on the surface as adults; the female becomes impregnated and the cycle is repeated.

Presentation

There is often intense itching, mainly of the hands, wrists and feet. The itching is particularly bad between the fingers where reddish spots (frequently with blood crusts, secondary to scratching) are seen.

Treatment

Because of the ease with which scabies is transmitted by close contact, treatment has to involve the whole family. The agents used are: Benzyl Benzoate, Crotamiton, Lindane, Malathion, or Monosulfiram.

SCHOOL REFUSAL

School refusal, or school phobia, arises when a child, otherwise physically well, is unable to go to school or experiences great difficulty in getting there. Instead of attending school, the child remains at home in a state of emotional distress and, at the same time, makes no attempt to conceal the problem. Parents of children who refuse to go to school always express concern and are usually fully aware of the problem.

School refusal has to be distinguished from truancy which usually occurs without the knowledge of the parents. The truant does not stay at home, but tends to wander the streets with other truants.

A further group of truants or 'pseudo' school refusers are those who stay off school with the collusion of their parents. Many of these children are from areas of social deprivation, frequently with parents who themselves found school unrewarding. Occasionally an agoraphobic mother, afraid to venture outside alone, will keep her daughter off school so that she will have company to go shopping. Often this type of sanctioning will be denied by the mother. A mother who has recently had a new baby will, at times, keep a daughter home to assist her. Another cause of 'pseudo' school refusal occurs in a family where the mother derives satisfaction from caring for a sick, dependent child and hence prolongs the convalescence considerably.

Normal children are occasionally reluctant to go to school in the first few years and a small number of them remain so throughout their school careers.

School refusal usually occurs in teenagers, and is unaffected by social class and gender, and has no relationship to intelligence or educational attainment. The onset of school refusal is often gradual, taking a few weeks to become established. During this time, there is a slow build-up of emotional upset at school time. Less frequently, the onset may be quite abrupt without any apparent underlying cause. Often, some event or series of events occurs prior to the initial problem which precipitated the onset of school refusal. These events may be:

- an incident at school relating to school work;
- an incident at school relating to relationship with peers;
- an illness necessitating absence from school;
- a holiday;
- moving from a small school to a larger one;
- moving classes;
- death of a relative or a pet;
- loss of a friend who moves away;
- victimisation or bullying.

Presentation

Although the child may rise early in preparation for school, as the time to depart approaches there is increasing anxiety and fearfulness. This anxiety manifests itself with acute physical symptoms and may result in any of the following:

- nausea;
- vomiting and anorexia;
- abdominal pain and diarrhoea;
- frequency of urination;
- pallor;
- headaches;
- trembling.

At times the symptoms are so severe that they may well mimic a physical illness – the so-called masquerade syndrome. If this is the case, the parents may well feel obliged to keep the child home from school. What sometimes confuses the picture is that the child may also demonstrate quite severe emotional problems, becoming obstinate, sulky, abusive and aggressive. At times, the child shows a quarrelsome dependency at home, alternating between panic and defiance. Other features, such as depression, tearfulness, hysteria, hypochondriasis and obsession may also be present.

Parental Attitudes

Often a child will be unduly dependent on his/her mother due to the mother being over-protective of the child. The child ends to cling, the parent becomes anxious and, as a result is often ineffective in the situation. The child often appears timid to observers, but is wilful and demanding at home and may well dominate the parent by becoming more aggressive. Much of the child's behaviour may be due to a separation anxiety.

Parental support may be lacking because the parent feels that the child has an actual illness, or that the school is, in some way, responsible for the situation.

Action at School

1   Steps should be taken to ascertain if any specific problems exist in the child's school environment. The assessment should include their academic progress, and the relationship with teaching staff, peers and friends. The possibility of victimisation or bullying should always be considered.
2   The attitude of the teacher towards the child and parents at the early stages is of the utmost importance, since initial reluctance to attend school can quite easily be turned to frank refusal.
3   There should be early involvement of the educational pyschologist and also the educational welfare officer. Referral for full psychiatric assessment and advice may also be necessary.

Treatment

A treatment plan should be worked out with the child and family and should involve the teacher. The manner in which the child is to return to school should be decided and if necessary, a suitable cover story prepared to explain the long absence. Plans should be instituted to recover any lost academic grades and for the child to catch up with the class notes to remove one of the areas of anxiety. Home tuition, as such, runs the risk of sanctioning absence.

It is felt by many that there should be an immediate return to school, with the parents and staff adopting a firm and consistent approach towards the child. For younger children, however, it may be necessary for their return to school to be more gradual. In the first instance, for example, it may be necessary for the child to be accompanied to school for a few days. Home visits by the teacher, or by some of the child's school friends prior to the planned return, might also be helpful. At times, parents may have to be reminded of their legal responsibilities before the child attends school.

If any particular problem or activity precipitated the initial refusal, then this should be solved or avoided. Occasionally, it may be necessary to place the child in a less demanding educational environment, for example, the use of a special unit as a 'half way house' between home and school by which attendances at school can be gradually increased.

In view of the emotional problems and occasionally the neuroses that sometimes accompany school refusal, it may be necessary to use psychotherapy, family therapy and behaviour modification.

SICKLE CELL DISEASE

This is one of a group of inherited blood diseases which cause anaemia, episodes of severe pain and infection. The most common and severe is sickle cell anaemia; other types are haemoglobin S-C disease and sickle B-thalassaemia which are less severe.

Prevalence

In the United Kingdom, sickle cell anaemia occurs more commonly in children of African or West Indian descent, and the incidence is about 1 in 400. It can also occur in children from the Eastern Mediterranean, India, Pakistan and the Middle East.

Cause

The defect present is sickle cell disease occurs in the protein haemoglobin found in the red blood cells. Haemoglobin is responsible for the transportation of oxygen to the tissues. It is a complex, coiled protein of which there are about 300 different types. The haemoglobin found in sickle cell disease has one wrong aminoacid substituted in the protein chain and this results in the haemoglobin behaving abnormally.

Normal adult haemoglobin (Hb A) is inherited from both parents – Hb AA. In sickle cell trait, one parent passes on sickle haemoglobin (Hb S) and the other normal haemoglobin (Hb A) resulting in Hb SA. Sickle cell trait does not cause an illness, but is a carrier state. About 1 in 10 children of African or West Indian descent have sickle cell trait. A child who receives sickle haemoglobin from both parents (Hb SS) has sickle cell anaemia.

When normal haemoglobin loses oxygen in the tissues, the red blood cells maintain their normal elastic shape which allows them to squeeze undamaged through the smaller blood vessels. However, when abnormal haemoglobin in sickle cell anaemia loses oxygen, it forms long crystals which change the round red cells into a sickle shape. These type of red cells are more rigid, thinner and longer than normal ones, and tend to block the smaller blood vessels. This is known as sickling. Most of the symptoms that occur are due to this phenomenon.

Presentation

Children with sickle cell disease may have certain recognisable features which can be obvious to the teacher. These are:

Anaemia
Almost every child with sickle cell disease has anaemia. The child may therefore appear pale, may be listless and tired and may have some degree of breathlessness. Many children, however, have no symptoms and are able to cope well.

Jaundice
Many children will be jaundiced – recognised by a yellowing of the whites of the eyes. The jaundice is due to excessive breakdown of the red cells with consequent increase in bile pigment in the tissues. The presence of jaundice does not mean that the child has hepatitis, or any other liver disease.

Infections
Children with sickle cell disease are very susceptible to infections, particularly pneumonia, meningitis and infections of the blood (septicaemia). Most take Penicillin daily to prevent infections occurring.

Urination
Most children with this disease need to pass urine frequently during the day. This is because they need to drink plenty of liquids to keep their blood from becoming too concentrated and hence prevent sickling from occurring. An adequate fluid intake is more important during hot weather, particularly after exercise.

Nose bleeds
Nose bleeds occur commonly in children with sickle cell disease but, although troublesome, they are rarely dangerous.

Pain

Pain occurs when normal blood flow in the smaller vessels becomes obstructed due to sickling of the red blood cells. The pain may be very severe and occurs most often in the arms and the legs. This may be accompanied, in some children, with swelling of the hands and feet and, occasionally, swelling of the joints. Pain may arise in other parts of the body, such as the chest, back, or abdomen. Occasionally, these painful crises are accompanied by a temperature.

Acute Problems

In the event of the following occurrences, the parents should be advised immediately and/or action taken to seek medical advice:

1 Any sudden increase in the degree of jaundice – which may indicate sickling in the liver.
2 A temperature of over 38°C (100.4°F) may be due to a bacterial infection and could be serious.
3 Diarrhoea and vomiting which could result in rapid loss of fluids, particularly in a young child and could lead to a painful crisis.
4 The onset of severe unexplained pain.

Before help is available, the child should be made comfortable and kept warm on a couch. Reassurance, comfort and a relaxing atmosphere is important, particularly if the child has pain, since panic and fear can make a crisis worse. Fluids, such as water, squash or milk should be given, at least a glassful every hour. Fizzy drinks should be avoided.

Prevention of Problems

Since anxieties regarding school work and examinations are thought to affect adversely the frequency of crises, the child requires considerable support and encouragement with studies. School work should be sent home for completion and during long absences, home tuition might be necessary.

Infections

Any rise in temperature should be reported to the school nurse or to the parents. The parents should be encouraged to give the necessary preventive antibiotic prescribed and any vitamins (e.g. folic acid), and should be encouraged to ensure that the child receives the full course of immunisation against infectious diseases.

Warmth

Ensure that the child is always warm and dry. Hot showering after exercise in the cold or swimming prevents chilling and reduces the risk of problems. A rapid change of temperature from a warm room to a cold outside environment should be avoided unless the child has adequate warm clothing.

School Work

Sickle cell disease has, apart from rare occasions, no effect on a child's intelligence. However, the child's schoolwork may be affected by listlessness and tiredness because of anaemia, by discomfort and occasional pain and by periods of absence from school.

Physical Activity

A child with sickle cell disease should be encouraged to participate in as much normal physical exercise in school as the condition allows. However, cross country running and outdoor games in cold or wet weather should be avoided. In some children the spleen may be enlarged and, if so, direct contact sports such as rugby and judo should be avoided. Under-water swimming which involves holding the breath should also be avoided.

Children with this disease should not be forced to take part in strenuous activity if they feel that it will bring on a painful crisis or breathlessness. As mentioned previously, warm showers after swimming or outdoor games are important.

Normal outings with the school on day trips should present no special problems if the precautions mentioned above are taken. School holidays such as skiing and trips requiring air travel should be discussed with the child's doctor.

See also   Thalassaemia

SPASTICITY – *see* Cerebral Palsy

SPEECH DEFECTS

By the time children are five years of age and most have started school, about 70% have normal speech and language development. About 20% have a minimal problem with the pronunciation of one or two letters and about 8% have some defect of articulation. After a year or two in school, there is usually some progressive maturity of speech and by the age of seven years, 95% have normal speech. About 4% continue to have articulation problems, 4% weak pronunciation of occasional letters and 1% are unintelligible.

DISORDER OF RHYTHM

During stages of early speech development most children have some hesitancy in the fluency of their speech. This hesitancy occasionally persists in the form of stammering or stuttering, which characteristically occurs at the beginning of sentences, the beginning of certain words, or words starting with certain letters. The defect is very common in young children but as they mature and gain confidence, it generally disappears. Some children, however, have presistent stammering and require help both in the classroom and with speech therapy.

DISORDER OF ARTICULATION

Disorders of articulation are very common in young children and interfere with their clarity of pronunciation. There may be substitutions of letters e.g. 'd' for 't' in 'whose dat dere' instead of 'whose that there' or 'k' for 't' in 'kekle' instead of 'kettle'. Certain letter substitutions give rise to lisping e.g. 'th' for 's' in 'yeth' instead of 'yes' and 'v' for 'r' in 'vobin' or 'vound' instead of 'robin' or 'round'. Another form of articulation disorder occurs by deletion of certain letters and occasionally words e.g. 'he go opital' instead of 'he goes to the hospital' or 'I go cool' instead of 'I go to school'.

Many of these defects are persistence of immature speech and as the child socialises in school and matures, so the speech becomes normal.

Causes

1. **Normal** – delayed maturity of speech which with time and increased self-confidence, becomes normal.
2. **Hearing defect** – some children, as a result of defective hearing, are unable to distinguish sounds clearly and hence, mispronounce words.
3. **Family history** – some families have a history of delayed speech or of speech disorders.
4. **Parents' speech** – children, at least initially, have a tendency to copy the articulation of their parents, not only with respect to their accents, but also with respect to diction. It is valuable, therefore, to talk to the parents of a child with a speech problem to ascertain their own speech pattern.
5. **Medical problems** – speech defects and delay are common in children who are mentally retarded. In some children with cerebral palsy there may be considerable problems of articulation because of a lack of coordination of the muscles required for speech. This is known as dysarthria. (See cerebral palsy)
6. **Emotional immaturity** – some children have a degree of emotional delay and with this, there may be an articulation disorder, the nature being the persistence of 'baby talk' with letter substitutions and deletions.
7. **Psychological causes** – various suggestions have been made regarding the possibility of psychological factors being the underlying cause of speech defects (e.g. insecurity, anxiety, separation, sibling rivalry, emotional abuse etc.). There is very little ground to substantiate this but children with established speech defects frequently lack confidence and their defect is likely to become temporarily worse if they are excited or stressed in any way.

Action by the Teacher

1. Speech defects which are encountered in the child's first year or so in school, and which are minimal, should be ignored since the majority of children develop normal speech.

2   Do *not* correct or point out the child's defect, particularly in front of the class as this leads to further lack of confidence.
3   *Do* encourage and praise the child for any effort at communication since this promotes self-confidence and more participation.
4   The child should only take part in reading aloud and answering questions in front of the class if willing. Reading aloud in twos and threes may be encouraged until the child gains sufficient confidence.
5   Singing, either in groups or individually, has helped many children overcome speech disorders, particularly stammering. Joining in puppet work may also be helpful.
6   Parents of children with severe or persistent speech defects should be advised to have the child's hearing tested and have an assessment carried out by a speech therapist.
7   If a child is undergoing treatment by a speech therapist, advice should be sought by the teacher regarding aspects of treatment that can be encouraged in school.

LANGUAGE DISORDER

A small percentage of children not only have difficulty in producing sounds, but also in producing phrases and sentences, and as a result have poor language expression. This is known as expressive aphasia or, if this is a milder form, dysphasia.

These children frequently have other associated problems such as hearing defects, perceptual problems and general educational difficulties. They require referral for detailed assessment and treatment.

STOMACH ACHE – *see* Abdominal Pain

THALASSAEMIA

Thalassaemia is the name given to a group of inherited anaemias which occur as a result of abnormal haemoglobin.

Cause

Normal haemoglobin, found in the red blood cell, is a complex coiled protein. It is responsible for the transportation of oxygen from the lungs to the tissues and carbon dioxide from the tissues to the lungs. The structure of haemoglobin is made up of a number of chemicals (amino-acids) joined together to form chains. Normal haemoglobin has four such chains, two with 141 amino-acids called alpha chains and two with 146 amino-acids called beta chains.

The defect in thalassaemia is the result of a reduced number of these essential amino-acid chains. A reduced number of alpha chains (141 amino-acids) gives rise to alpha thalassaemia and a reduced number of beta chains (146 amino-acids) to beta thalassaemia.

Thalassaemia is transmitted because of a genetic defect present in one or both parents. If the defect is passed by one parent it is known as heterozygous, and from both parents it is known as homozygous.

A genetic defect of beta chain formation transmitted from one parent (heterozygous) produces a condition known as thalassaemia minor. Transmission of the defect from both parents (homozygous) produces the condition thalassaemia major which is also known as Mediterranean anaemia or Cooley's anaemia. A genetic defect in the formation of alpha chain formation transmitted from one parent (heterozygous) produces a mild anaemia. Transmission from both parents (homozygous) produces a severe anaemia which causes foetal death.

THALASSAEMIA MAJOR (MEDITERRANEAN ANAEMIA, COOLEY'S ANAEMIA)

Presentation

This produces a severe, chronic anaemia which becomes evident in early infancy. Characteristically, children with this condition have a poor rate of growth and are small in stature. Bone changes occur making fractures more common, and the effect on the bones of the skull produces prominence of the forehead and a tendency towards protruding teeth. Children are generally very pale and have an enlargement of the liver and the spleen. There is delayed puberty, with absent or little evidence of sexual development. In girls menstrual periods may be absent, or, the amount of blood loss minimal.

Treatment

The long-term treatment of this condition is by means of repeated blood transfusions. Unfortunately, the treatment may, in itself, produce problems since frequent transfusions result in an excess of iron from the transfused blood being deposited in the child's tissues. However, the risk of this happening is now reduced by simultaneously using an intravenous preparation that binds iron – hence rendering it harmless.

Problems in School

1 The child's physical activity may be limited because of tiredness and breathlessness as a result of chronic anaemia. The extent of activity will have to be gauged by the extent of the illness and the child's ability to participate.
2 Body contact sports such as soccer, rugby, judo and boxing should be avoided, particularly if there is enlargement of the spleen.
3 As in sickle cell anaemia, crises may occur if the child develops any infections and similar precautions have to be

taken (*see* Sickle Cell Disease). Occasionally it is necessary to remove the spleen by surgery and this may increase the susceptibility to infections. Children who have had their spleen removed take daily antibiotic treatment to reduce this risk.

Since the aim of treatment is to maintain the child's haemoglobin at a near normal level it is necessary for the child to undergo blood transfusions every 4 to 6 weeks. This usually means missing 1 to 2 days of school.

THALASSAEMIA MINOR

This condition is due to the heterozygous form of beta thalassaemia and produces a mild anaemia which is compatable with normal life and life expectancy.

HETEROZYGOUS ALPHA THALASSAEMIA

This produces an anaemia which may be slightly more severe than thalassaemia minor but not as severe as thalassaemia major.

See also   Sickle Cell Disease

VERRUCAS (PLANTAR WARTS)

Verrucas are caused by a virus which is transmitted by direct contact from floors in and around swimming pools and showers. They are painful, deep-seated nodules found on the soles of the feet.

Prevention is by adequate use of disinfected foot baths before and after swimming. Any child who has a verruca should be referred for treatment and in the meantime should wear a tight rubber stocking whilst using the swimming pool or showers, to prevent the spread of infection.

VISUAL DEFECTS

Defective eyesight and squints are the most common conditions recorded during medical examinations in schools.

Prevalence

In a survey carried out in 1971, 3 million school children were examined for eye problems. Approximately 130 000 needed treatment because of defective vision; a further 240 000 needed further observation. In addition, approximately 22 000 required treatment for squints and a further 21 000 required observation for the same problem.

This survey showed that there was an overall incidence rate of 50 per 1000 children requiring treatment and an additional 87 per 1000 children requiring further observation.

Presentation

The onset of defective vision is often gradual. One of the first signs is a decline in school progress, errors in copying work from the blackboard and a reluctance to read aloud or, in fact, to read at all. The child has to hold reading books close to the face and adopts a similar position when writing. The handwriting becomes untidy and writing on lines becomes increasingly more difficult.

It may be noted that the child also becomes clumsy in the classroom, or during play in ball games and there may be a tendency to become accident-prone. Frowning and blinking may be present and occasionally there may be an abnormal head posture when reading.

SQUINT

Squint, strabismus, or cross eye is a common disorder estimated to occur in about 5% of children. It occurs as a result of a misalignment of the axis of the eye. The most common type is that which causes the eye to turn inwards – a convergent squint. Failure to recognise this and to treat it could result in a life-long visual defect of the affected eye. Unfortunately, if a squint remains undiagnosed after the age of two years, it is unlikely that damage to the eyesight can be prevented.

The initial visual problems caused by a squint is double vision or diplopia. Children compensate for this by tilting the head to one side, hence bringing both eyes into alignment. Occasionally, depending on which eye muscle is affected, the child may tilt the head backwards or forwards. An awareness of such head posture as a presenting feature of squint could possibly result in early recognition of an underlying problem. A squint is often only noticed, initially, if a child is tired or unwell.

The treatment of the condition is firstly to restore any refractive error by the wearing of glasses, if necessary, accompanied by covering or obstructing the vision of one eye. Finally, the axis of the eye is realigned by altering surgically the tension in one or more of the external eye muscles.

SHORT SIGHTEDNESS OR MYOPIA

In this condition the length of the eye is too long and the image from a distant object consequently falls short of the retina. A child with this condition can see clearly objects which are close at hand but not those further away, with resulting difficulty in seeing what is written on the blackboard. In view of the fact that vision may be normal in the early years, it is important to take note of a child who gradually complains of not being able to see the writing on the blackboard.

LONG SIGHTEDNESS OR HYPERMETROPIA

Children with this condition have a shorter eye than normal and images of objects fall behind the retina. This has the opposite effect to short sightedness and results in the child not being able to see close objects, such as writing on books, but seeing distant objects clearly.

Both are termed errors of refraction and are corrected by the wearing of suitable spectacles.

Action by the Teacher

If a teacher suspects that a child has a visual problem, the parents should be informed and advised to seek an optical assessment immediately. In the interest of the child, the teacher should ensure that such advice has been acted upon, and if possible should request the results of such examinations. If a visual defect is established it is important to ensure that the child wears any prescribed glasses when in school. It may be necessary for the child to sit at the front of the class; if one eye has very poor vision, the child should sit with the good eye towards the middle of the classroom. A good reading light may be an additional necessity for some children.

SEVERE VISUAL PROBLEMS

At the present time, there are approximately 1200 blind and 2300 partially sighted children receiving education in special schools or units in the United Kingdom. Approximately 25% of these children will have suffered an additional handicap sufficient to require special education. A further 25% will have less serious associated defects but ones which will cause learning difficulties. Physical handicap and educational subnormality are the two most commonly found associated handicaps in children who are severely visually impaired. Others are epilepsy, behavioural problems, speech difficulty and hearing defects.

The more common causes of severe visual handicap are as follows:

1 Injury to one or both eyes with damage and scarring of the cornea and/or lens.
2 Congenital opacity of the lens and cataract.
3 Surgical removal of the eye due to tumour or severe infection with bacteria or protozoa.
4 Defective development of the eye.
5 Optic atrophy – loss of visual function of the optic nerve.
6 Albinism.
7 Disease of the retina.

Special appliances may be required for children with severe

visual problems. These may be magnifying glasses, large print books, or a Visuotek system which magnifies books on to a television screen.

BLINDNESS

Children who are blind fall into two causative groups – those who are born blind, and those who become blind later on in childhood. In the former group, there may be associated handicaps which preclude ordinary school placement. Although some children who are born blind have no other handicap, they may require, for normal development, an intensive programme of stimulation in the first four to five years. Such a programme may require education at a residential school for the blind.

Children who become blind during their school life should be encouraged to stay in an ordinary school, if at all possible.

Advice regarding education and aids for the blind and partially sighted children can be obtained from the Royal National Institute for the Blind, who have regional advisers for this purpose.

WHOOPING COUGH

Whooping cough presents with paroxysms of coughing which last uninterrupted for about 2 to 3 minutes. During such paroxysms, the child's face becomes red or even blue. The spasm is followed by a noisy, forcible, inhalation of air which produces the characteristic whoop, although this is not always necessarily present. The onset of the coughing stage is preceeded by a runny nose.

Transmission

By direct contact, or by droplet spread or indirectly, by contact with freshly contaminated articles from an infected child.

Incubation Period

From 5 to 21 days but usually within 10 days.

Infectious Period

This is greatest in the stage preceding the onset of coughing and the child remains infectious up to about 4 weeks after the onset of symptoms. The infectious period may be reduced if the child receives certain specific antibiotics.

USEFUL ADDRESSES

AFASIC (Association for all Speech Impaired Children), 346 Central Market, Smithfield, London EC1 9NH. Tel: 01-236 3632/6487.

British Diabetic Association, 10 Queen Anne Street, London W1M OBD. Tel: 01-323 1531.

British Epilepsy Association, Crowthorne House, New Wokingham Road, Wokingham, Berkshire RG11 3AY. Tel: 0734 587345.

British Dyslexia Association, Church Lane, Peppard, Oxon RG9 5JN. Tel: 0491 7699.

Centre on Environment for the Handicapped, Great Smith Street, London W1. Tel: 01-222 7980. (Bibliography and information sheet on play and play equipment for handicapped children.)

Cystic Fibrosis Research Trust, 5 Blyth Road, Bromley, Kent BR1 3RS. Tel: 01-464 7211.

Department of Education and Science, Elisabeth House, 39 York Road, London SE1 7PH. Tel: 01-934 9000.

Disabled Living Foundation, 380-384 Harrow Road, London W9 2HU. Tel: 01-289 6111 (Lists and advice on aids, publications and addresses of organisations for the disabled.)

Dyslexia Institute (Information Centre), 133 Gresham Road, Staines, Middlesex PW18 2AJ. Tel: 0784 59498.

Health Education Authority, 78 New Oxford Street, London WC1 1AH. Tel: 01-631 0930.

Haemophilia Society, PO Box 9, 16 Trinity Street, London SE1 1DE. Tel: 01-407 1010.

Muscular Dystrophy Group of Great Britain, Nattrass House, 35 Macauley Road, Clapham, London SW4 0QP. Tel: 01-720 8055.

National Toy Libraries Association, 68 Churchway, London NW1 1LT. Tel. 01-387 9592.

Partially Sighted Society, 40 Wordsworth Street, Hove, East Sussex BN3 5BH. Tel: 0273 736053.

POSSUM Controls Ltd, Middlegreen Trading Estate, Middlegreen Road, Slough, Berkshire SL3 6DF. Tel: 0753 79234.

Royal National Institute for the Blind, 224 Great Portland Street, London WIN 6AA. Tel: 01-388 1266.

Royal National Institute for the Deaf (Information Directory), 105 Gower Street, London WC1E 6AH. Tel: 01-387 8033.

Sickle Cell Society, c/o Brent Community Health Council, 16 High Street, Harlesden, London NW10 4LX. Tel: 01-459 1292.

Spastics Society, Advice Service, 16 Fitzroy Square, London WIP 5HQ. Tel: 01-387 9571.

Spastics Society Publications, The Librarian, Spastic Society, 12 Park Crescent, London WIN 4EQ. Tel: 01-636 5020.

Visually Handicapped Advisory Service, Disabled Living Foundation, 380-384 Harrow Road, London W9 2HU. Tel: 01-289 6111.

Welsh Office Information Division, Cathays Park, Cardiff CF1 3NQ. Tel: 0222 825111.

FURTHER READING

DEPARTMENT OF EDUCATION AND SCIENCE (1978) *Special Educational Needs* (Warnock Report). London: HMSO.

GRIFFITHS, M. AND RUSSELL, P. (1985) *Working Together with Handicapped Children: Guidelines for Parents and Professionals.* London: Souvenir Press Ltd.

HMSO (1976) *Court Report: Fit for the Future.* London: HMSO.

JEFFREE, D. M.; MCCONKEY, R. AND HEWSON, S. (1981) *Teaching the Handicapped Child.* London: Souvenir Press Ltd.

LENNOX, W. G. (1960) *Epilepsy and Related Disorders.* London: J. and A. Churchill.

LIBRARY ASSOCIATION (1978) *Reading for the Visually Handicapped.* London.

MALE, J. AND THOMPSON, C. (1985) *The Educational Implications of Disability.* London: The Royal Association for Disability and Rehabilitation.

MILES, T. R. (1974) *The Dyslexic Clinic* (p. 128). London: Priory Press.

PRIOR, M. R. AND GRIFFIN, M. W. (1985) *Hyperactivity: Diagnosis and Management.* London: William Heinemann Medical Books.

WATLING, R. (1973) *Identification of the Larger Fungi* (p. 114). Amersham: Hulton Educational Publications.

WOODS, G. E. (1983) *Handicapped Children in the Community.* Bristol: John Wright and Sons Ltd.

INDEX OF SYMPTOMS